The Common Sense Guide to Weight Loss: A Carnivore-Paleo Approach

Dedication

This book is dedicated to everyone who has ever felt the frustration of yo-yo dieting and the weight of unrealistic expectations. It's for those who have battled with their bodies and felt defeated by fad diets that promise quick fixes but deliver only temporary results. This is for the busy professionals, the overwhelmed parents, and anyone who longs for a simple, sustainable, and enjoyable path to a healthier weight and a happier life. This is dedicated to the power of consistency, the importance of self-compassion, and the unwavering belief in your ability to transform your health. This journey is not just about the number on the scale; it's about reclaiming your energy, boosting your confidence, and feeling truly empowered in your own skin. May this book serve as your unwavering companion, guiding you toward a healthier, happier, and more fulfilling life. This is for you, the reader, who is brave enough to embark on this life-changing journey and create a sustainable, healthy future for yourself. May this guide equip you with the knowledge and tools needed to conquer your weight, not just for today, but for a lifetime of well-being.

Preface

For years, the weight-loss industry has been awash with complicated diets, restrictive eating plans, and unrealistic promises. Countless individuals have fallen prey to these quick-fix solutions, only to find themselves back at square one, often feeling more discouraged than ever. This book offers a different approach—a refreshing alternative that emphasizes simplicity, sustainability, and genuine well-being. This book takes the best of two impactful approaches, the Carnivore and Paleo diets, carefully combining them to create a practical and flexible strategy that aligns with your unique lifestyle and needs. This is not about deprivation; it's about nourishing your body with nutrient-dense foods that satiate you, energize you, and support your overall health. This book provides a straightforward path toward achieving sustainable weight loss, focusing on building healthy habits that will last a lifetime. Forget the restrictive rules and complicated calculations. Instead, embrace a sensible approach that combines the power of real food, mindful eating, and a supportive community. I encourage you to approach this journey with self-compassion, celebrate your progress, and never give up on your goals. Your health deserves this effort. The simple approach outlined in this book prioritizes sustainable changes that create lasting results, rather than relying on quick fixes that lead to inevitable disappointment. This is a journey of empowerment, discovery, and lasting transformation—and I am thrilled to guide you along the way.

Introduction

Are you tired of fad diets that leave you feeling deprived and discouraged? Do you long for a sustainable approach to weight loss that doesn't involve complicated rules or restrictive eating patterns? If so, you've come to the right place. This book presents a practical and empowering guide to achieving sustainable weight loss by combining elements of the Carnivore and Paleo diets. This hybrid approach leverages the benefits of both: the enhanced satiety and reduced inflammation often associated with the Carnivore diet, and the emphasis on nutrient-dense, whole foods found in the Paleo diet. The principles of this approach are founded on consuming primarily animal-based products—meat, fish, poultry, and eggs—while optionally incorporating healthy fats, some vegetables, nuts and seeds, depending on individual tolerances. This allows for greater flexibility and customization compared to the stricter protocols of each individual diet. The emphasis is on real food, not processed foods, grains, or added sugars—ingredients that often sabotage weight-loss efforts. This book goes beyond simply listing foods to avoid; it equips you with the knowledge and practical strategies to succeed. You'll learn how to create simple, delicious meals, manage social situations, build sustainable habits, and incorporate enjoyable exercise into your routine. This isn't just about losing weight; it's about transforming your relationship with food, building a healthier lifestyle, and achieving lasting well-being. Get ready to embark on a journey towards a healthier, happier, and more energetic you. Prepare to learn how to nourish your body, fuel your vitality, and cultivate a positive and sustainable relationship with both food and fitness. This book is your comprehensive guide to successfully navigate the process, ensuring long-term success and a happier, healthier lifestyle. Let's begin!

Calorie Balance Explained

Weight loss, at its core, is a matter of energy balance. This seemingly simple concept is often misunderstood, leading to frustration and ineffective dieting strategies. Understanding the science behind it is crucial for achieving sustainable weight loss and maintaining a healthy lifestyle. The fundamental principle is straightforward: to lose weight, you need to expend more energy (calories) than you consume. This energy balance is governed by three primary components: your basal metabolic rate (BMR), your activity levels, and the thermic effect of food (TEF).

Your basal metabolic rate (BMR) represents the number of calories your body burns at rest to maintain basic bodily functions like breathing, blood circulation, and organ function. Your BMR is influenced by several factors, including your age, gender, body composition (muscle mass versus fat mass), genetics, and even your current hormonal balance. Generally, individuals with higher muscle mass have a higher BMR because muscles require more energy to maintain than fat tissue. Age also plays a significant role; as we age, our BMR tends to decrease, meaning we burn fewer calories at rest. This is one of the reasons why weight management can become more challenging with age. It's important to note that BMR is not a fixed number; it can fluctuate slightly based on various factors, including stress levels and sleep quality.

Understanding your BMR is essential because it forms the foundation of your daily caloric needs. However, your BMR alone doesn't tell the whole story. Your activity level significantly impacts your overall energy expenditure. This encompasses all physical activity you engage in throughout the day, from walking to work, cleaning your house, engaging in formal exercise, and even fidgeting. The more active you are, the more calories you burn. The intensity and duration of the activity also play a crucial role; a vigorous workout burns significantly more calories than a leisurely stroll. Accurate tracking of your activity level, whether through wearable fitness trackers or meticulous journaling, allows for a more precise calculation of your daily caloric expenditure. This precision helps in creating a tailored weight loss plan.

Finally, the thermic effect of food (TEF) refers to the calories your body burns in the process of digesting, absorbing, and metabolizing the food you consume. This process is not always passive; it requires energy. Protein has a higher TEF compared to carbohydrates and fats. This means that consuming a diet rich in protein can boost your metabolism and contribute to a slightly higher daily caloric expenditure. However, TEF accounts for a relatively small percentage of your total daily energy expenditure, usually around 10%, so it's not the primary driver of significant weight loss. While it plays a supplementary role, focusing on protein-rich foods offers numerous other benefits, including increased satiety and muscle preservation, aspects crucial for sustainable weight loss.

Calculating your total daily energy expenditure (TDEE) requires combining your BMR, activity level, and TEF. Online calculators can provide estimates of your TDEE, but remember that these are just approximations. Individual factors influence these numbers. To achieve weight loss, you need to create a calorie deficit. This means consuming fewer calories than your body expends. The size of this deficit determines the rate of weight loss. A moderate calorie deficit of 500-750 calories per day is generally recommended for sustainable weight loss, resulting in a loss of approximately

1-1.5 pounds per week. A more aggressive deficit might lead to quicker weight loss initially, but it's often unsustainable in the long run and may lead to nutrient deficiencies or muscle loss.

Creating a sustainable calorie deficit isn't about drastically restricting your food intake or starving yourself. It's about making smart choices, focusing on nutrient-dense whole foods, and finding an eating pattern that works for you long-term. The Carnivore-Paleo approach, which emphasizes whole, unprocessed foods, is designed to promote satiety and reduce cravings, making it easier to manage calorie intake without feeling deprived. This approach tends to naturally support a calorie deficit due to the high protein and fat content of the foods, leaving you feeling full and satisfied. The focus on whole, minimally processed foods also supports a healthier metabolic environment.

Furthermore, it's crucial to remember that weight loss is not solely a numerical game; the quality of the calories you consume matters. While a calorie deficit is essential, prioritizing nutrient density is equally important. Nutrient density refers to the amount of nutrients per calorie. Whole, unprocessed foods, especially those found in the Carnivore-Paleo framework, are far more nutrient-dense than highly processed foods. A diet rich in these nutrients supports overall health, improves metabolic function, and can even help regulate appetite, making it easier to maintain a calorie deficit. This is where the Carnivore-Paleo approach shines; it inherently prioritizes nutrient-rich whole foods.

The detrimental effects of neglecting nutrient density, even while maintaining a calorie deficit, should not be underestimated. Cutting calories drastically without considering nutrient intake can lead to significant deficiencies. This can result in fatigue, weakness, impaired immune function, and even metabolic disturbances. These deficiencies can ultimately hinder your weight loss efforts and negatively impact your overall health. Choosing whole, unprocessed foods ensures that your body receives all the necessary vitamins, minerals, and antioxidants, supporting optimal health and aiding in sustained weight loss.

Moreover, it's essential to understand that the human body isn't a simple equation. Individual metabolic responses vary significantly. While the calorie deficit is fundamental, factors such as genetics, gut microbiome composition, hormonal balance, and stress levels all play a role. What works
effectively for one person might not be as effective for another. A sustainable approach recognizes this variability and encourages flexibility and adaptation based on individual needs and responses.

Remember, sustainable weight loss is a marathon, not a sprint. It requires a holistic approach that incorporates not just diet but also regular physical activity, sufficient sleep, and effective stress management. The information presented here provides a scientific foundation to guide your weight loss journey. The following chapters will delve deeper into the Carnivore-Paleo approach, providing practical strategies, meal plans, and recipes to help you achieve your weight loss goals in a healthy and sustainable way. The goal isn't just weight loss, but lasting health and well-being.

The Role of Macronutrients in Weight Management

The success of any weight-loss strategy hinges on a nuanced understanding of macronutrients—protein, fat, and carbohydrates—and their individual roles in energy balance, satiety, and overall health. While the Carnivore-Paleo approach emphasizes whole, unprocessed foods, understanding how these macronutrients interact is crucial for optimizing your weight loss journey and maintaining long-term success.

Let's begin with protein, often hailed as the king of macronutrients for weight management. Protein possesses a uniquely high thermic effect, meaning your body expends more energy digesting and processing it compared to carbohydrates or fats. This increased energy expenditure contributes to a slightly higher caloric deficit, aiding in weight loss. Moreover, protein is incredibly satiating. It promotes feelings of fullness and reduces cravings, helping you adhere to your caloric goals without constant hunger pangs. This is particularly important when embarking on a weight-loss journey, as consistent hunger can often derail even the most determined individuals. Think of protein as your ally in the battle against hunger-induced snacking.

The importance of adequate protein intake extends beyond satiety; it's vital for preserving lean muscle mass during weight loss. When you're in a caloric deficit, your body needs a readily available source of amino acids to prevent muscle breakdown. Without sufficient protein, your body may start using muscle tissue for energy, slowing your metabolism and potentially making it harder to lose weight in the long run. This is why strength training, coupled with a high-protein diet, is a powerful combination for successful weight management. Aim to consume a gram of protein per pound of lean body mass daily, or even slightly more, to support muscle preservation and enhance the overall effectiveness of your weight loss plan. Excellent sources of protein within the Carnivore-Paleo framework include lean meats (beef, poultry, lamb), fatty fish (salmon, tuna, mackerel), eggs, and organ meats (liver, kidney). These foods offer not only protein but also essential vitamins and minerals.

Next, let's address the role of fat. Often demonized in the past, dietary fat has undergone a significant rehabilitation in recent years, and rightfully so. Healthy fats are essential for hormone production, cell function, and nutrient absorption. Furthermore, they too contribute to satiety, keeping you feeling full and satisfied between meals. Unlike carbohydrates, fats are not easily converted into stored body fat, and they play a crucial role in regulating appetite hormones such as leptin and ghrelin, helping to curb your cravings. However, the type of fat matters. Prioritize healthy fats like those found in avocados, nuts (in moderation if following a stricter Carnivore approach), seeds (similar moderation caveats apply), olive oil, and fatty fish. These fats are rich in monounsaturated and polyunsaturated fatty acids, which offer numerous health benefits beyond just weight management. Limit saturated and trans fats found in processed foods, fried foods, and some animal products. These types of fats should be kept to a minimum within the Carnivore-Paleo approach. Focusing on healthy fats is essential not only for weight loss but for overall metabolic health.

Now, let's discuss carbohydrates. The Carnivore-Paleo approach minimizes carbohydrate intake, opting instead for a predominantly protein and fat-based diet. This is not to say that carbohydrates are inherently "bad"; rather, the emphasis is on reducing the intake of refined carbohydrates, added sugars, and processed grains that are often devoid of nutritional value and contribute to blood sugar spikes and crashes. These spikes and crashes often lead to increased hunger, cravings, and ultimately, weight gain. The approach isn't about completely eliminating carbohydrates, but rather selecting nutrient-dense sources like certain vegetables and fruits, while substantially reducing or eliminating refined grains, sugars, and processed foods.

Within the context of a Carnivore-Paleo approach, the role of carbohydrates is minimized, and the focus is on the satiating and metabolic benefits of protein and fat. The body's preference for using fat and protein as energy sources, when these are plentiful, helps to regulate blood sugar levels and prevent the roller-coaster effect associated with high carbohydrate intake. For many, this reduction in carbohydrate intake leads to significant weight loss as the body naturally utilizes stored fat for energy. However, it's important to note that individual responses vary, and some individuals may experience better results with a slightly higher intake of non-starchy vegetables, providing additional fiber and micronutrients.

It's crucial to understand that the Carnivore-Paleo approach isn't a rigid, one-size-fits-all system. The level of carbohydrate restriction should be personalized based on individual metabolic needs, activity levels, and personal preferences. If you find yourself experiencing excessive fatigue or other adverse effects from significantly limiting carbohydrates, it may be worthwhile consulting a registered dietitian or healthcare professional to adjust your macronutrient ratios. The goal is to find a sustainable balance that optimizes your weight loss progress without compromising your overall well-being.

It is also important to consider the quality of carbohydrates you do consume. Non-starchy vegetables like leafy greens, broccoli, and cauliflower are excellent sources of fiber, vitamins, and minerals and can be included in moderation even in a stricter Carnivore diet. These add bulk to the diet promoting satiety without a significant impact on blood sugar.

Remember that successful weight management isn't solely about macronutrient ratios; it's a holistic approach that encompasses several factors. Sufficient hydration, adequate sleep, effective stress management, and regular physical activity all play crucial roles in optimizing your body's ability to lose weight and maintain a healthy weight. Think of the macronutrient balance as one important piece of a larger puzzle.

In conclusion, understanding the roles of protein, fat, and carbohydrates is fundamental to achieving sustainable weight loss within the Carnivore-Paleo framework. Prioritizing high-quality protein for satiety and muscle preservation, incorporating healthy fats for satiety and metabolic health, and minimizing refined carbohydrates and added sugars are key strategies. However, remember that personalizing your approach is vital for success. Consulting with a healthcare professional or registered dietitian can help you determine the optimal macronutrient balance for your individual needs and ensure that your weight-loss journey is both effective and safe. Remember, sustainable weight loss is a journey, not a race, and consistent, informed choices are crucial for long-term success and improved overall health and well-being. The goal isn't just to lose weight, but to cultivate healthier habits that will serve you for years to come. By focusing on nutrient-dense, whole foods and incorporating regular physical activity and stress management, you can achieve sustainable weight loss and a healthier, happier life. This approach isn't about restriction, but about nourishing your body with the best possible foods to support your overall health and well-being. The long-term rewards of a healthy lifestyle far outweigh the short-term sacrifices involved in making these changes. Remember to be patient, persistent, and celebrate your progress along the way!

Debunking Weight Loss Myths and Misconceptions

The journey to achieving and maintaining a healthy weight is often fraught with misinformation and misleading shortcuts. Many individuals embark on this path armed with myths and misconceptions, hindering their progress and potentially harming their health. Let's address some of the most pervasive fallacies surrounding weight loss, offering evidence-based counterarguments to empower you with accurate information and a realistic approach.

One of the most persistent myths is that low-carbohydrate diets are inherently dangerous. The fear often centers on concerns about nutritional deficiencies, metabolic acidosis, and the dreaded "keto flu." While it's true that a poorly planned low-carb diet can lead to some of these issues, a well-structured approach, such as the Carnivore-Paleo diet we've discussed, actively mitigates these risks. The key is to focus on nutrient-dense, whole foods rather than relying on processed low-carb alternatives. A diet rich in animal protein, healthy fats, and, where appropriate, select non-starchy vegetables, provides a balanced nutritional profile, ensuring adequate intake of essential vitamins and minerals.

The concern about metabolic acidosis, a feared consequence of low-carbohydrate diets, is largely unfounded in the context of a balanced, whole-foods approach. While it's true that the body produces ketones when carbohydrates are limited, this process is a natural metabolic adaptation, not a dangerous condition. Furthermore, the kidneys and lungs work efficiently to maintain a healthy acid-base balance, preventing the development of harmful acidosis. The "keto flu," characterized by fatigue, headache, and nausea, is typically a temporary adjustment period as the body adapts to using fat as its primary fuel source. These symptoms are often alleviated by increasing water and electrolyte intake, including sodium, potassium, and magnesium. This phase passes as your body adjusts.

Another common misconception revolves around the belief that only cardiovascular exercise contributes to weight loss. While cardio undoubtedly plays a role in burning calories and improving cardiovascular health, it's only part of the equation. Strength training, for example, is crucial for building and preserving muscle mass, which increases your resting metabolic rate. This means your body burns more calories even at rest, significantly aiding weight loss and maintenance. Moreover, strength training improves body composition, leading to a more toned and sculpted physique. This aspect often provides a sense of accomplishment and motivates individuals to continue their fitness journey.

The belief that spot reduction—targeting fat loss in specific areas—is possible is another widely held misconception. Your body burns fat proportionally throughout the whole body, not just in areas where you exercise. While localized exercise strengthens muscles in specific areas, it doesn't preferentially burn fat in those regions. For overall fat reduction, a combination of diet and exercise, addressing your overall caloric balance, is essential. Focusing on a whole-body approach leads to more sustainable and healthy weight loss.

Many believe that rapid weight loss is synonymous with effective weight loss. The truth is, rapid weight loss often leads to muscle loss, nutrient deficiencies, and, importantly, a higher chance of weight regain. Sustainable weight loss is a gradual process aimed at making lasting lifestyle changes. Aiming for a consistent, healthy rate of weight loss (1-2 pounds per week) ensures that you are losing fat and not muscle. This slow and steady method improves your chances of maintaining your new weight in the long run. Quick fixes are temporary, and focusing on long-term, sustainable habits is crucial for long-term success.

Another pervasive misconception is that weight loss is solely determined by willpower. While willpower plays a role, it's not the sole determinant of success. Underlying factors such as genetics, metabolism, hormones, stress levels, sleep quality, and gut health all contribute significantly to your weight. Ignoring these elements can lead to frustration and failure. A holistic approach, recognizing and addressing these factors, improves your chances of achieving your weight goals. This includes stress-management techniques, prioritization of sleep, and potential interventions to address any underlying hormonal imbalances or gut issues.

A further misconception is that all calories are created equal. This ignores the significant difference between nutrient-dense, whole foods and processed, calorie-dense foods. For example, 100 calories from broccoli will provide numerous nutrients and fill you up, whereas 100 calories from a sugary drink provide few nutrients and contribute little to satiety. Prioritizing whole, unprocessed foods within a caloric deficit is far more effective and satisfying than relying on restrictive low-calorie diets filled with processed foods. The latter approach often leads to cravings and ultimately unsustainable weight loss.

Similarly, the misconception that "you can eat anything as long as you're in a calorie deficit" is dangerously misleading. While caloric deficit is important, focusing only on calories ignores the quality of those calories. A diet consisting of processed foods, even within a caloric deficit, can lead to poor health, low energy levels, and a compromised immune system. It can also lead to nutritional deficiencies that can affect various aspects of health, including hormone balance, metabolism, and overall well-being.

Many believe that certain foods are "fattening" or "weight-loss friendly." The concept of classifying foods as "good" or "bad" is an oversimplification. There's no single magic food or food group that guarantees weight loss. Your success hinges on making balanced and informed choices within the context of a balanced diet that prioritizes whole, unprocessed foods. This means integrating various types of nutrient-rich food while limiting or avoiding processed foods, sugary drinks, and excessive refined carbohydrates.

Some think that once you reach your goal weight, you can revert to your old eating habits. This is perhaps the most dangerous misconception. Sustained weight loss requires permanent changes in lifestyle and dietary habits. The moment you return to old patterns, the weight is likely to creep back. It is a fundamental change in how you fuel your body, not a temporary fix.

Finally, remember that setbacks are inevitable on any weight-loss journey. Don't let a slip-up derail your progress. A single indulgent meal or a week of less-than-ideal choices doesn't negate your previous successes. Learn from the experience, adjust your approach as needed, and get back on track. This is a marathon, not a sprint, and consistency over time is paramount.

By understanding these debunked myths and misconceptions, you can embark on your weight-loss journey with a more accurate and realistic perspective, increasing your chances of achieving your goals sustainably and improving your overall health and well-being. Remember, the Carnivore-Paleo approach, with its emphasis on nutrient-dense, whole foods, provides a robust framework to support this journey. However, individual needs vary, and consulting with a registered dietitian or healthcare professional is always recommended to personalize your plan and ensure it's safe and effective for you.

Setting Realistic Goals and Expectations

Building a sustainable weight-loss journey isn't about drastic, unsustainable changes; it's about making gradual, consistent shifts that integrate seamlessly into your life. The key lies in setting realistic goals and expectations, understanding that lasting weight management is a marathon, not a sprint. This section will guide you through this crucial step, helping you craft a plan that's both ambitious and attainable.

One of the biggest pitfalls in weight loss is setting goals that are simply too ambitious. Aiming for a rapid weight loss of several pounds a week might seem appealing initially, promising quick results. However, this approach is often unsustainable and can lead to burnout, frustration, and ultimately, failure. Rapid weight loss frequently involves drastic calorie restriction, which can negatively impact your metabolism, energy levels, and overall well-being. It can also lead to muscle loss, rather than fat loss, which is counterproductive to long-term health and fitness. Your body needs time to adapt to the changes you are implementing, and pushing it too hard too quickly will only backfire.

Instead of focusing on a specific number on the scale, consider setting smaller, more achievable goals. For instance, rather than aiming to lose 20 pounds in two months, start by setting a goal of losing 1-2 pounds per week. This slower, more gradual approach allows your body to adjust gradually, minimizing stress and maximizing the chances of long-term success. Remember, even small changes can lead to significant results over time. A consistent loss of 1-2 pounds per week translates to a substantial weight loss of 4-8 pounds per month, which adds up considerably over several months.

Another effective strategy is to focus on non-scale victories. These are the positive changes that occur beyond the numbers on the scale. For example, you might focus on improving your energy levels, increasing your strength, improving your sleep quality, fitting into your clothes more comfortably, or feeling more confident and energetic. Tracking these non-scale victories helps reinforce the positive changes you're making, even if the scale doesn't always reflect your progress immediately. Weight loss is a complex process, and the number on the scale can fluctuate due to various factors like water retention, hormonal changes, and even bowel movements. Focusing solely on the number on the scale can be incredibly discouraging, leading to feelings of failure, even when real progress is being made. Celebrating non-scale victories helps maintain motivation and celebrate the positive steps being taken.

To set realistic goals, consider your current lifestyle, activity levels, and dietary habits. Honest self-assessment is critical. If you currently lead a sedentary lifestyle and consume a highly processed diet, aiming for a significant weight loss in a short timeframe might not be realistic. Start by setting smaller, more achievable goals, such as incorporating 30 minutes of moderate-intensity exercise most days of the week and gradually reducing processed foods from your diet. As you achieve these smaller goals, you can gradually increase the intensity and duration of your exercise and further refine your diet, setting progressively challenging goals as you build momentum and confidence.

Progress tracking is another crucial aspect of setting realistic expectations. It provides valuable insights into your progress and helps you stay motivated. Tracking your weight, measurements, and food intake allows you to identify patterns and make necessary adjustments to your plan. However, it's essential to track your progress in a way that's sustainable and doesn't add unnecessary stress. Frequent weighing can lead to unnecessary anxiety and discouragement, particularly if the numbers don't always reflect the desired outcome. Aim for weekly weigh-ins, always at the same time of day to ensure consistency. Avoid daily weigh-ins to prevent emotional distress and minimize any discouraging fluctuations.

Instead of solely relying on the scale, consider tracking your measurements (waist circumference, hip circumference, etc.). These measurements provide a more comprehensive picture of your progress, as muscle gain may not be reflected on the scale. Measuring your waist circumference is especially important, as it's a strong indicator of visceral fat—the unhealthy fat stored around your organs. Tracking your body measurements in addition to your weight allows you to better understand the changes happening in your body and to monitor progress, regardless of the scale.

Photography can also be a helpful tool in visualizing your progress. Taking monthly progress pictures, while maintaining consistent lighting and posing, can help you visualize your body composition changes. A full-length photo taken in front of a mirror each month can be a great way to document the changes in your body shape and size that may not be readily apparent on the scale. It provides a visual representation of your progress over time, creating a motivating incentive for continued effort.

Consider keeping a food journal to track your daily food intake. This doesn't need to be excessively detailed; a simple record of what you ate, when you ate it, and approximately how much can provide valuable insights. A food journal allows you to identify patterns in your eating habits, such as snacking tendencies or times when you are more likely to overeat. Becoming aware of these patterns is essential to address them constructively and develop healthier strategies.

In addition to tracking your weight, measurements, and food intake, consider tracking your overall well-being. This could include factors such as sleep quality, stress levels, energy levels, and mood. Tracking these elements allows you to better understand how your weight-loss efforts impact your overall health and well-being, highlighting the importance of overall balance. If you notice an impact on these areas, it might be necessary to adjust your plan to ensure you are supporting your overall health, not just your weight-loss goal.

Remember, setting realistic goals and expectations is crucial for long-term success. It's a journey of gradual progress, not a race against time. By focusing on small, achievable steps, tracking your progress effectively, and celebrating both big and small wins, you'll create a sustainable approach that promotes not only weight loss, but also your overall health and well-being. Be patient with yourself; consistent effort, not instant gratification, is the key to lasting results. Embrace the process and focus on the positive changes you're making along the way. Remember to consult with your doctor or registered dietitian to personalize your plan and ensure it aligns with your individual needs and health status. They can provide valuable guidance and support to help you achieve your goals safely and effectively. Remember, the ultimate goal is not just weight loss, but the cultivation of a healthier, happier, and more energetic you.

Building a Support System for Success

Building a strong support system is paramount to achieving your weight loss goals and maintaining a healthy lifestyle long-term. The journey towards a healthier you is often challenging, filled with ups and downs, temptations, and moments of self-doubt. Having a network of supportive individuals can significantly increase your chances of success by providing encouragement, accountability, and a sense of community.

One of the most effective ways to build a support system is to connect with others who share similar goals. This could involve joining online forums, social media groups, or local support groups dedicated to healthy eating and weight management. These communities offer a space to share experiences, recipes, and tips, fostering a sense of camaraderie and mutual support. You can find encouragement when facing setbacks, celebrate successes together, and gain valuable insights from others' journeys. The collective experience can be incredibly powerful, reminding you that you are not alone in this process.

Online communities offer accessibility and convenience, particularly beneficial for those with busy schedules or geographical limitations. Many dedicated Facebook groups, subreddits, and online forums are devoted to the Paleo and Carnivore diets, offering support, recipes, and advice. However, be discerning when choosing an online community. Look for groups that promote a positive and supportive environment, avoiding those that engage in negativity, body shaming, or promote unhealthy practices. It is essential to find a community that aligns with your values and dietary approach.

Offline support can be equally beneficial. Consider joining a fitness class, participating in a walking group, or even simply inviting a friend or family member to join you on your health journey. Sharing your goals with someone close to you can hold you accountable and provide much-needed encouragement. Having a friend to exercise with, for instance, can make workouts more enjoyable and sustainable. Sharing meals prepared according to the Carnivore-Paleo principles can simplify meal planning and provide a sense of shared experience.

Family support can be particularly crucial. Openly communicating your goals with your family and requesting their understanding and support is vital. This might involve explaining the rationale behind your dietary choices and seeking their cooperation in avoiding tempting foods at home. Family dinners can be adapted to fit the Carnivore-Paleo principles, creating opportunities for shared meals and bonding. However, it's essential to approach this with sensitivity and understanding. Family members may need time to adjust to the changes, and your approach should be one of education and gentle persuasion rather than imposition.

Beyond direct support groups, consider seeking professional guidance from a registered dietitian or a health coach specializing in low-carbohydrate diets. These professionals can provide personalized advice, create tailored meal plans, and offer ongoing support and accountability. Their expertise can address any concerns or challenges you might encounter along the way, ensuring that your weight loss efforts are safe and effective. Regular check-ins with a professional can help you stay motivated and address any obstacles that may arise.

Remember, building a supportive network isn't just about finding people who understand your dietary choices; it's also about cultivating relationships built on mutual respect, understanding, and support. Choose individuals who encourage your progress, celebrate your successes, and offer a compassionate ear during challenging times. This could involve friends, family, colleagues, or even online acquaintances. The key is to find individuals who understand and genuinely support your journey.

Accountability is another crucial element of a successful weight loss plan. This involves having someone to check in with regularly, to share your progress (and setbacks), and to help keep you motivated. This could be a friend, family member, or a professional such as a health coach. Regular check-ins provide an opportunity to discuss any challenges you're facing, brainstorm solutions, and stay on track. Sharing your progress also promotes self-reflection and allows you to identify areas where you might need additional support or adjustments to your plan.

Some effective strategies for incorporating accountability into your weight loss journey include:

Regular check-ins with a support partner:
Schedule regular meetings, either in person or virtually, with a friend or family member who supports your goals. Discuss your progress, challenges, and upcoming plans.

Joining a weight loss challenge or program:
Participating in a structured program with a defined timeline, goals, and support system can provide external accountability and motivation.

Using a weight loss app or tracking tool:
Many apps offer features to track your progress, set goals, and connect with

others on similar journeys, providing a form of built-in accountability.

Working with a health professional:
A registered dietitian or health coach can provide ongoing support, monitor your progress, and make necessary adjustments to your plan as you progress.

Beyond formal accountability partnerships, building a broader network of support is equally valuable. Sharing your journey with others—even casually—can provide a sense of belonging and encouragement. Talking about your goals and progress with colleagues, friends, and family can help reinforce your commitment and gain moral support.

However, remember that seeking support is not a sign of weakness but rather a strategic approach to increasing your chances of success. The journey towards weight loss is rarely a solo endeavor. Surrounding yourself with a strong network of support provides resilience, encouragement, and the resources needed to navigate challenges and celebrate milestones along the way.

Remember to choose your support system wisely. While encouragement is essential, it's equally crucial to distance yourself from individuals who might undermine your progress through negativity, discouragement, or conflicting advice. It's about surrounding yourself with individuals who genuinely want to see you thrive and succeed.

Building a robust support system is an ongoing process, not a one-time event. As your journey progresses, your needs and support structure might change. Be open to adapting your support network, adding new connections, and refining existing relationships as you navigate the various stages of your weight loss journey. Cultivating a supportive and understanding environment is a crucial investment in your long-term success and well-being.

In conclusion, the weight loss journey is significantly enhanced by a well-constructed support system. This isn't simply about having people who understand your dietary choices, but a network that offers encouragement, accountability, and a shared sense of community. By carefully cultivating this network – through online communities, in-person support groups, family, friends, and professional guidance – you will significantly increase the likelihood of achieving your weight loss goals and, more importantly, maintaining a healthy lifestyle for years to come. Remember, this isn't a sprint; it's a marathon, and having the right support team by your side makes all the difference. Embrace the opportunity to connect, share, and learn from others on this enriching journey toward a healthier and happier you.

Core Principles of the Carnivore Diet

The carnivore diet, in its purest form, is remarkably simple: it consists solely of animal products. This includes various cuts of red meat (beef, lamb, pork), poultry (chicken, turkey), fish and shellfish, and eggs. Organ meats, like liver and kidney, are also frequently included, as they are exceptionally nutrient-dense. Dairy products, while technically animal-derived, are often excluded due to their carbohydrate content, particularly lactose. However, some individuals on the carnivore diet may incorporate them in moderation, depending on their individual tolerance and goals.

The core principle underlying the carnivore diet is the elimination of plant-based foods entirely. This includes fruits, vegetables, nuts, seeds, legumes, and grains – essentially everything that falls outside the realm of animal products. The rationale behind this stark restriction stems from several key beliefs. One is the belief that many individuals experience improved digestive health and reduced inflammation by removing plant compounds like lectins, phytic acid, and various carbohydrates which some believe can be difficult for the human digestive system to process efficiently. Another key belief centers around the argument that our ancestral diet consisted predominantly of animal products, implying a biological predisposition towards a more carnivorous lifestyle. While there is significant debate surrounding the exact nature of our ancestral diet, the carnivore diet proponents suggest that this dietary approach aligns more closely with our evolutionary history.

One of the frequently touted benefits of the carnivore diet is enhanced satiety. The high protein and fat content of animal products creates a feeling of fullness that can last for several hours, potentially reducing cravings and minimizing the need for frequent snacking. Many adherents report significant weight loss on this diet, attributed to the naturally low carbohydrate content, encouraging the body to utilize stored fat for energy. This metabolic shift is often associated with ketosis, a state where the body burns fat for fuel instead of glucose.

However, the carnivore diet is not without its potential drawbacks and limitations. A primary concern is the potential for nutrient deficiencies. While animal products are rich in many essential nutrients, they may lack sufficient amounts of certain vitamins and minerals commonly found in plant-based foods. Vitamin C, for instance, is often cited as a potential concern, as it's abundant in fruits and vegetables but absent in meat. Similarly, fiber, crucial for healthy gut function, is entirely absent from a strictly carnivorous diet. While some argue that the body can obtain sufficient vitamin C from the liver and other organ meats and that beneficial gut bacteria can thrive on the byproducts of meat digestion, others contend that supplementation may be necessary to address these potential gaps. The lack of fiber is a particularly critical consideration, as it plays a vital role in gut health and bowel regularity.

Furthermore, the extremely restrictive nature of the carnivore diet can pose challenges for long-term adherence. The limited variety of food choices can lead to monotony and make it difficult to maintain the diet over an extended period. For individuals who enjoy culinary diversity or find pleasure in preparing and consuming a wide range of foods, the strict limitations of the carnivore diet might prove unsustainable. Social situations and eating out can also be a significant obstacle, as many restaurants do not cater to such a highly specific dietary approach. Preparing meals that meet the requirements can be time-consuming, and purchasing and storing large quantities of meat and eggs is a considerable undertaking.

The potential impact on kidney health is another area of concern for some experts. The high protein intake associated with the carnivore diet could place added stress on the kidneys, especially for individuals with pre-existing conditions. However, this concern is often debated, with some studies indicating no significant negative effect on kidney function in healthy individuals consuming a high-protein diet. Nevertheless, individuals with kidney issues should certainly consult their physician before considering the carnivore diet.

Another aspect to consider is the potential for high saturated fat intake. While saturated fat is not inherently harmful in moderation, a diet heavily reliant on red meat can lead to a significant increase in saturated fat consumption, potentially elevating cholesterol levels in some individuals. However, this remains a complex and often debated topic in the nutritional field. Some research suggests that saturated fat may not be as detrimental to cholesterol levels as previously believed, while other studies maintain that restricting saturated fat remains important for cardiovascular health. Again, personalized advice from a healthcare professional is crucial.

The potential for increased uric acid levels is another concern. Animal products are relatively high in purines, which the body metabolizes into uric acid. Elevated uric acid levels can contribute to gout, a painful inflammatory condition affecting the joints. Individuals with a history of gout should exercise caution and closely monitor their uric acid levels while on a carnivore diet. Regular blood tests are highly recommended to monitor various health markers, including kidney function, cholesterol levels, and uric acid levels.

In summary, the carnivore diet presents a unique approach to nutrition, promising significant benefits such as weight loss, enhanced satiety, and reduced inflammation for some individuals. However, its highly restrictive nature and the potential for nutrient deficiencies necessitate careful consideration and monitoring. It's crucial to weigh the potential benefits against the potential risks and consult with a healthcare professional or registered dietitian to determine if the carnivore diet is appropriate and safe for you. Regular blood tests are essential to monitor your health markers and to address any potential nutrient imbalances promptly. While the diet might be suitable for some, it may not be appropriate or sustainable for others, underscoring the importance of personalized dietary choices.

Core Principles of the Paleo Diet

The Paleo diet, often referred to as the "caveman diet," offers a compelling alternative to modern processed food-laden lifestyles. Its core principle revolves around mimicking the dietary habits of our Paleolithic ancestors, a time before the advent of agriculture and processed foods. This approach emphasizes consuming whole, unprocessed foods that were naturally available to our ancestors, focusing on nutrient density and minimizing the intake of foods believed to be detrimental to health.

The foundational premise of the Paleo diet rests on the assumption that our bodies are biologically adapted to the foods consumed by our ancestors over millennia. This implies that modern processed foods, refined sugars, grains, and legumes, which have only become prevalent in recent human history, may be incompatible with our evolved physiology. Proponents of the Paleo diet suggest that these foods contribute to chronic diseases such as obesity, type 2 diabetes, heart disease, and autoimmune disorders. By eliminating these potentially problematic foods and focusing on nutrient-rich alternatives, Paleo adherents aim to improve their overall health and well-being.

Central to the Paleo dietary framework is the concept of nutrient density. This refers to the concentration of essential vitamins, minerals, antioxidants, and other beneficial compounds relative to the caloric content of a food. Paleo-friendly foods, such as lean meats, wild-caught fish, fruits, and vegetables, are generally rich in these essential nutrients. Conversely, processed foods often contain high levels of calories but are low in essential nutrients, leading to a potential nutritional deficiency despite adequate calorie intake. Understanding nutrient density is key to making informed food choices. The emphasis isn't merely on calorie restriction but on choosing foods that provide maximum nutritional value for their calorie count, maximizing the body's ability to function optimally.

The Paleo diet allows for a wide range of foods, emphasizing those readily available to our ancestors. Meat, including beef, lamb, pork, poultry, and game, is a cornerstone of the diet, providing high-quality protein and essential fats. Fish and shellfish offer valuable omega-3 fatty acids and other nutrients. Eggs, another crucial element, are packed with protein, choline, and essential vitamins. Fruits and vegetables, providing a rich array of vitamins, minerals, fiber, and antioxidants, constitute a significant part of a well-rounded Paleo diet. Nuts and seeds, although not consumed in the quantities found in modern supermarkets, are permitted in moderation, contributing healthy fats and other beneficial compounds. The inclusion of these natural foods, with their complex nutrient profiles, differentiates the Paleo diet from many other restrictive approaches. This breadth of permissible foods helps to ensure satiety, minimize nutrient deficiencies, and ultimately promote adherence.

However, understanding what
not
to consume is just as crucial as knowing which foods are acceptable on the Paleo diet. The diet explicitly excludes a number of food groups that are commonly found in modern diets. Refined grains, such as white bread, pasta, and pastries, are off-limits due to their high glycemic index and low nutritional value.
Processed sugars, typically found in candy, soft drinks, and other sweet treats, are strictly avoided to minimize sugar spikes and crashes and prevent potential metabolic dysregulation. Legumes, such as beans, lentils, and peas, although nutritious in some respects, are excluded due to their potential to inhibit nutrient absorption and cause

digestive distress in some individuals. Processed foods, which contain refined sugars, unhealthy fats, artificial additives, and preservatives, are strictly avoided, emphasizing instead the consumption of whole, unprocessed alternatives. Dairy products are a point of contention among Paleo followers; some choose to exclude them altogether, while others incorporate them moderately, depending on individual tolerance. The exclusion of these foods is not solely based on caloric considerations but primarily stems from a belief that they negatively impact long-term health, contributing to inflammation and chronic disease.

It's important to emphasize that the Paleo diet isn't a one-size-fits-all approach. Individual needs and preferences must be carefully considered. For instance, individuals with certain allergies or sensitivities may need to make adjustments to accommodate their specific needs. Furthermore, while the underlying principle is based on ancestral eating patterns, the practicality of procuring and preparing foods exactly as our ancestors did is often challenging in modern society. A modern interpretation of the Paleo diet typically prioritizes whole, unprocessed foods readily available and affordable today. This modern adaptation avoids the unrealistic expectations of adhering strictly to a purely Paleolithic diet, allowing for greater accessibility and sustainability.

The benefits often attributed to following a Paleo diet are numerous, but it's crucial to remember that individual responses can vary considerably. Weight loss is commonly reported among individuals who switch to a Paleo-style of eating. This is often attributed to the increased consumption of protein and fiber, which can lead to greater satiety and reduced calorie intake. The emphasis on whole foods generally results in higher nutrient intake, which supports optimal metabolic function and can help regulate appetite.

Reduced inflammation is another frequently cited benefit. The elimination of processed foods, refined sugars, and other potentially inflammatory substances is believed to play a significant role in alleviating inflammation associated with chronic diseases. Improved blood sugar control is frequently observed in individuals following a Paleo diet, partly due to the low glycemic index of the permissible foods. This improved blood sugar regulation is particularly beneficial for those at risk of or already diagnosed with type 2 diabetes. Enhanced energy levels are also often reported, likely due to the increased nutrient intake and avoidance of blood sugar spikes and crashes.

However, potential drawbacks associated with the Paleo diet should also be addressed. Nutrient deficiencies can occur if the diet is not carefully planned. For example, if sufficient sources of calcium and vitamin D are not included, bone health may be compromised. Similar issues can arise if the diet is deficient in fiber or certain B vitamins. Strict adherence to a Paleo diet can also be expensive, particularly if relying heavily on organic and grass-fed meats. The restrictive nature of the diet can also make social events and dining out more challenging. Therefore, finding a balance between adhering to the principles of the diet and incorporating flexibility is often crucial for long-term success.

In summary, the Paleo diet offers a compelling framework for improving health and well-being through a focus on whole, unprocessed foods consumed by our ancestors. It emphasizes nutrient density, minimizing processed foods, refined sugars, and grains. While offering potential benefits such as weight loss, reduced inflammation, and improved blood sugar control, individuals should be mindful of potential pitfalls, including nutrient deficiencies and cost considerations. Careful planning and consultation with a registered dietitian or healthcare professional are recommended to ensure a balanced and sustainable approach. A flexible adaptation of the Paleo principles, rather than strict adherence to a purely Paleolithic diet, might be a more realistic and achievable long-term strategy for most individuals. The ultimate aim remains to prioritize long-term health and well-being over short-term results. Remember, the Paleo diet isn't a magic bullet; it's a lifestyle change that requires careful planning, thoughtful execution, and a commitment to understanding one's own individual needs and preferences.

A Synergistic Approach

The Paleo diet, with its emphasis on whole, unprocessed foods, provides a solid foundation for healthy eating. However, some find its breadth of permitted foods – fruits, vegetables, nuts, and seeds in addition to meats and fish –can be challenging to navigate, particularly when aiming for weight loss. This is where the synergistic power of combining elements of the Carnivore and Paleo diets comes into play. This hybrid approach offers a streamlined, highly satiating diet that simplifies meal planning while maximizing the potential for weight management and improved metabolic health.

The core concept lies in leveraging the best aspects of both diets. The Carnivore diet's extreme focus on animal products– meat, fish, poultry, and organ meats – offers unparalleled simplicity. It eliminates the guesswork associated with
carbohydrate counting and the potential for hidden sugars in seemingly healthy foods. This stark simplicity can be incredibly beneficial for individuals overwhelmed by the intricacies of food choices, especially those new to dietary changes. The high protein and fat content of a Carnivore diet promotes satiety, reducing cravings and making it easier to maintain a caloric deficit – a crucial element for successful weight loss. Furthermore, the absence of plant-based foods, often associated with inflammatory responses in some individuals, can lead to a reduction in inflammation, benefiting those with inflammatory conditions.

However, the exclusive focus on animal products within the Carnivore diet raises concerns regarding nutrient diversity. While animal products provide essential nutrients, relying solely on them might lead to deficiencies in certain vitamins, minerals, and phytonutrients found abundantly in plant-based foods. This is where the Paleo diet offers valuable supplementation. By selectively incorporating certain fruits, vegetables, nuts, and seeds, we can address these potential nutritional gaps while maintaining the core principles of a low-carbohydrate, high-protein, high-fat approach.

Choosing the "right" foods from both approaches is key. The emphasis should remain firmly on whole, unprocessed foods. This means avoiding processed meats, opting instead for grass-fed beef, wild-caught fish, and free-range poultry. Organ meats, often overlooked, should be considered a valuable source of essential nutrients, including vitamins A, B12, and various minerals. Eggs, particularly pasture-raised eggs, also hold a place of honor, providing a complete protein source along with vital nutrients.

When incorporating plant-based components from the Paleo framework, prioritize nutrient-dense options. Leafy green vegetables like spinach, kale, and collard greens are excellent sources of vitamins and minerals, offering essential micronutrients without significantly impacting blood sugar levels. Cruciferous vegetables such as broccoli and cauliflower are also beneficial, offering fiber and various phytochemicals. However, starchy vegetables like potatoes and sweet potatoes should be consumed sparingly, owing to their higher carbohydrate content.

The selection of fruits should also be thoughtful. Berries, known for their lower sugar content compared to other fruits, can provide antioxidants and fiber. However, it's important to consume berries in moderation. Nuts and seeds, like almonds, walnuts, and chia seeds, can add healthy fats, fiber, and essential nutrients. However, portion control is essential as they are relatively calorie-dense. The key here is to find a balance: adding sufficient amounts of these plant-based foods to optimize nutrient intake without significantly increasing carbohydrate intake and hindering weight loss progress.

This combined approach isn't about strict adherence to fixed ratios or proportions. It's about creating a personalized, sustainable diet that caters to individual needs and preferences. An individual's unique metabolic response, sensitivities, and overall health should guide the specific composition of this hybrid diet. For some, it might mean primarily focusing on animal products, with only a small amount of carefully selected plant foods to complement their nutrient intake. For others, a more balanced approach – perhaps 80% animal products and 20% carefully selected plant-based foods – might be more suitable.

The crucial element is listening to one's body. Pay attention to how different foods affect energy levels, satiety, digestion, and overall well-being. If certain foods cause digestive discomfort or contribute to unwanted weight fluctuations, they should be either limited or eliminated. Flexibility and adaptation are key. This isn't a rigid diet; it's a journey of discovering what works best for your body and your lifestyle.

Beyond the food choices, consistent hydration is paramount. Water plays a critical role in metabolic processes, aiding digestion and supporting overall bodily functions. Aim to drink plenty of water throughout the day. Herbal teas, unsweetened, can also be included as part of a healthy hydration strategy.

Regular physical activity is another vital component of successful weight management. The choice of exercise should be enjoyable and sustainable. Walking, strength training, and high-intensity interval training (HIIT) are all effective options. The aim is to incorporate regular physical activity into one's routine, enhancing cardiovascular health and boosting metabolism. Find activities you genuinely enjoy – this will make adhering to an exercise routine far more achievable in the long run.

Furthermore, prioritizing sleep is crucial. Sufficient sleep contributes to hormonal balance, regulating appetite and metabolism. Aim for 7-9 hours of quality sleep per night to support your weight loss goals and overall well-being.

Tracking progress is essential for maintaining motivation. This could involve regularly weighing yourself, measuring body fat percentage, or monitoring other health indicators relevant to your individual health goals. Seeing tangible results provides encouragement and motivation to stay on track.

Finally, fostering supportive relationships and cultivating a positive mindset play a significant role in successful weight management. Joining support groups, connecting with others who share similar goals, and seeking professional guidance can provide the encouragement and motivation needed to overcome challenges and achieve lasting success.

The Carnivore-Paleo hybrid approach is more than just a diet; it's a lifestyle shift that prioritizes nourishment, sustainability, and well-being. It empowers individuals to take control of their health, adopting a simple yet effective approach to weight management and improved metabolic health. Remember, this is a journey, not a race. Consistency, patience, and a focus on long-term sustainable habits are key to achieving lasting success and reaping the numerous health benefits this approach offers. By carefully selecting whole, unprocessed foods and listening to one's body, individuals can discover a personalized, enjoyable, and sustainable way to nourish themselves and achieve their health and weight management goals. Always consult with a healthcare professional or registered dietitian before making significant dietary changes, particularly if you have pre-existing health conditions. They can provide personalized guidance and address any specific concerns you might have. The focus should always remain on long-term health and well-being, not just short-term weight loss.

Addressing Potential Nutritional Concerns

The streamlined nature of the Carnivore-Paleo approach, while offering significant benefits in terms of weight management and satiety, necessitates a careful consideration of potential nutritional gaps. While the diet prioritizes nutrient-dense whole foods, certain vitamins and minerals may require closer attention to ensure optimal health. This isn't to say that deficiencies are inevitable; rather, a proactive and informed approach is essential. Let's examine some key areas.

One frequent concern revolves around Vitamin C. Unlike the Paleo diet, which allows for a wider variety of fruits and vegetables rich in Vitamin C, the Carnivore-Paleo approach significantly restricts plant-based foods. While organ meats like liver are excellent sources of Vitamin C, relying solely on these for sufficient intake might prove challenging for some. Therefore, supplementing Vitamin C is often recommended, particularly if you are rigorously adhering to a stricter version of the diet with minimal vegetable inclusion. The recommended daily allowance (RDA) varies depending on age and other factors, so consulting a healthcare professional to determine the appropriate dosage for your individual needs is paramount. They can help you find a high-quality supplement and monitor your levels through regular blood tests.

Fiber intake is another area demanding vigilance. Fiber, predominantly found in plant-based foods, plays a crucial role in digestive health, promoting regular bowel movements and maintaining a healthy gut microbiome. The reduced fiber intake associated with the Carnivore-Paleo approach could lead to constipation if not carefully managed. While some fiber can be obtained through consuming organ meats, the quantity is significantly less compared to a diet rich in fruits, vegetables, and whole grains. Strategic incorporation of low-carbohydrate, high-fiber vegetables like leafy greens (in moderation) can help mitigate this. However, individuals may still need to consider a supplemental fiber source, such as psyllium husk or a similar product, to ensure adequate intake. Remember to increase fiber intake gradually to avoid digestive discomfort.

Beyond Vitamin C and fiber, other micronutrients warrant monitoring. For instance, the diet's emphasis on animal products may lead to higher saturated fat intake. While saturated fat isn't inherently harmful in moderation, it's crucial to ensure balance and monitor cholesterol levels through regular blood tests. These tests, along with complete blood counts (CBCs) and comprehensive metabolic panels, are essential for assessing overall nutritional status and identifying any potential deficiencies or imbalances. Regular monitoring allows for proactive adjustments to the diet or supplementation strategy, ensuring that this approach remains a sustainable and healthy choice.

The importance of regular blood testing cannot be overstated. It's not merely a precautionary measure; it's an integral part of responsible dietary management. Routine blood tests provide invaluable insights into your body's nutritional status, allowing for early detection and correction of any imbalances. Ideally, you should consult your doctor or a registered dietitian to establish a testing schedule tailored to your individual needs and health history. They can advise on the specific tests necessary, interpret the results
accurately, and provide tailored recommendations based on your unique circumstances. This proactive approach significantly enhances the safety and effectiveness of the Carnivore-Paleo approach.

Some may argue that relying on blood tests for nutritional guidance is overly cautious or even unnecessary. However, it's important to remember that individual responses to dietary changes can vary significantly. Genetic predisposition, existing health conditions, medication interactions, and even gut microbiome composition can influence how your body absorbs and utilizes nutrients. Therefore, relying solely on general guidelines or anecdotal evidence is insufficient. Regular blood testing offers a personalized, objective assessment that removes the guesswork, empowering you to make informed decisions about your diet and supplement regimen.

Let's discuss the practical aspects of incorporating supplements and addressing potential nutrient deficiencies within the Carnivore-Paleo framework. It's crucial to choose high-quality supplements from reputable manufacturers, as the quality and purity of supplements can significantly impact their effectiveness and safety. Look for third-party tested products to ensure they meet the labeled claims and are free from contaminants. Furthermore, it is wise to start with lower dosages and gradually increase them as needed, always under the guidance of a healthcare professional. This minimizes the risk of adverse reactions and allows your body to adjust to the new additions.

Supplementing shouldn't be seen as a replacement for a well-planned diet. Rather, it's a complementary strategy to fill potential nutritional gaps and optimize overall health. While supplements can be beneficial, they should never replace the core principle of the Carnivore-Paleo approach: consuming nutrient-dense whole foods. Prioritizing high-quality animal products, including organ meats, remains paramount for optimal health. Supplements are simply a tool to support, not replace, a well-structured diet.

The choice of supplements depends entirely on your individual needs, as determined by regular blood tests and consultation with your healthcare provider. However, some commonly recommended supplements for individuals following the Carnivore-Paleo approach include Vitamin C, magnesium, and omega-3 fatty acids. Vitamin C, as discussed earlier, is essential for immune function and overall health, particularly when fruit and vegetable intake is restricted. Magnesium plays a vital role in various bodily functions, including muscle and nerve function, blood sugar control, and blood pressure regulation. Omega-3 fatty acids, predominantly found in fatty fish, are vital for brain health, heart health, and reducing inflammation. While the Carnivore-Paleo approach provides some omega-3s, supplementation might be necessary for individuals who don't consume sufficient amounts of fatty fish.

Addressing potential nutrient deficiencies within the Carnivore-Paleo approach isn't about resorting to a complex regimen of multiple supplements. Instead, it's about taking a proactive and informed approach, using regular blood tests to guide your choices. This personalized strategy prioritizes your specific needs, ensuring that this dietary approach aligns with your long-term health goals. Remember, this dietary pattern is intended to promote health and well-being; it is not a one-size-fits-all solution.

Beyond the specific micronutrients, there are broader considerations for maintaining overall health while following a Carnivore-Paleo diet. Hydration is paramount; ensure you are consistently drinking plenty of water throughout the day. Sufficient hydration supports numerous bodily functions, including digestion, nutrient absorption, and temperature regulation. Regular physical activity is equally important, contributing to overall well-being, weight management, and mental health. Choose activities that you enjoy and that fit your lifestyle, whether it's brisk walking, strength training, or something else entirely. Prioritize sleep; adequate rest is essential for hormone regulation, muscle recovery, and overall health.

Finally, and perhaps most importantly, listen to your body. Pay attention to how you feel, both physically and mentally. Adjust your diet and lifestyle as needed to accommodate your individual needs and preferences. This is a journey, not a race, and sustainable changes are more important than rapid results. The Carnivore-Paleo approach should empower you to make informed choices and take control of your health and well-being. Remember that this dietary pattern is a tool, and its effectiveness hinges on thoughtful planning, regular monitoring, and a commitment to long-term health. The role of consistent communication with your healthcare provider remains crucial throughout this process. By working collaboratively, you can develop a personalized approach that supports both your weight management goals and your overall well-being.

A Holistic Approach

The Carnivore-Paleo approach isn't merely a diet; it's a philosophy centered around nourishing your body with whole, unprocessed foods and fostering a mindful relationship with your eating habits. This holistic perspective extends beyond simply shedding pounds; it's about cultivating a sustainable lifestyle that promotes long-term health and well-being. At its core, this approach emphasizes the power of nutrient-dense foods to fuel your body optimally, reducing inflammation, and improving overall vitality.

The emphasis on whole foods is paramount. This means prioritizing foods in their most natural state, minimizing or eliminating processed ingredients, additives, and refined carbohydrates. Animal products—meat, poultry, fish, and eggs—form the foundation, providing high-quality protein, essential fats, and a range of micronutrients. The optional inclusion of certain vegetables, nuts, and seeds further enhances the nutritional profile, offering a broader spectrum of vitamins, minerals, and antioxidants. However, the core principle remains the avoidance of processed foods, grains, and added sugars, which are often associated with
inflammation, weight gain, and chronic diseases.

Nutrient timing, while not a strict rule, plays a supporting role within this philosophy. Consuming nutrient-dense meals and snacks throughout the day helps maintain stable energy levels, reduces cravings, and prevents overeating. This isn't about following rigid schedules; instead, it's about consciously choosing foods that provide sustained energy and satiety, preventing the energy crashes and hunger pangs often associated with processed food consumption.

Understanding your body's hunger and fullness cues becomes crucial. This mindful approach to eating promotes a healthier relationship with food, moving away from emotional eating and toward intuitive eating practices.

Beyond the immediate benefits of weight management, the Carnivore-Paleo philosophy emphasizes the long-term advantages for overall health. By reducing inflammation, improving gut health, and optimizing nutrient intake, this dietary approach can contribute to a reduced risk of several chronic diseases. Many individuals find that this way of eating improves their energy levels, enhances their sleep quality, and sharpens their cognitive function. These improvements aren't solely attributed to weight loss; they reflect the positive impact of consuming nutrient-dense whole foods and eliminating processed foods and sugar.

The gut microbiome, often overlooked in traditional weight-loss approaches, plays a pivotal role in the success of the Carnivore-Paleo philosophy. The elimination of processed foods, particularly those high in refined carbohydrates and added sugars, can significantly benefit the balance of gut bacteria. An imbalance in gut microbiota is linked to various health issues, including weight gain, inflammation, and impaired immunity. By focusing on whole, unprocessed foods, the Carnivore-Paleo approach encourages the growth of beneficial bacteria, which aids digestion, strengthens the immune system, and may contribute to weight management. The high protein intake, also a central feature, is believed to improve gut barrier function and reduce intestinal permeability, a factor contributing to inflammation and various health problems.

Furthermore, the mental and emotional aspects are inextricably linked to the success of any dietary approach, and the Carnivore-Paleo philosophy is no exception. Mindful eating—paying attention to your hunger and fullness cues, savoring your meals, and eating without distractions—plays a crucial role in promoting a healthy relationship with food. Stress management is also important. Chronic stress can lead to overeating and hinder weight-loss efforts. Incorporating stress-reducing activities, such as meditation, yoga, or spending time in nature, complements the dietary approach, fostering both physical and mental well-being. The reduction in inflammation, a common consequence of this way of eating, can also significantly impact mood, reducing anxiety and improving overall mental clarity. The elimination of sugar fluctuations, a common trigger for mood swings, is another key contributor to improved mental well-being.

The simplicity of the Carnivore-Paleo approach is another crucial aspect of its long-term sustainability. Unlike many fad diets that impose restrictive rules and complex meal plans, this approach focuses on making simple, informed choices. By emphasizing whole foods, it naturally reduces the likelihood of cravings and the need for constant willpower. The relative ease of meal preparation also contributes to its long-term practicality, avoiding the time and effort often associated with more complicated diets. This is achieved by focusing on straightforward cooking methods and minimizing the need for extensive recipe research or specialized ingredients. This straightforward approach reduces the mental burden often associated with dieting, facilitating long-term adherence. It empowers individuals to take control of their health without feeling overwhelmed or constantly battling cravings.

The concept of a 'clean plate' and the pressure to finish everything on your plate often contributes to overeating and can be counterproductive to weight management goals. The Carnivore-Paleo philosophy encourages intuitive eating, which means listening to your body's signals of hunger and fullness. Instead of forcing yourself to eat everything served, pay attention to your body's cues and stop eating when you feel satisfied, not stuffed. This prevents overconsumption, supports a healthy relationship with food, and ultimately contributes to weight management. It is a crucial element in building a long-term healthy relationship with food and avoiding the pitfalls of restrictive dieting.

However, it is crucial to acknowledge that the Carnivore-Paleo approach isn't a one-size-fits-all solution. Individual needs and tolerances vary considerably. While it offers significant benefits for many, some individuals may require adjustments or supplements to meet their specific nutritional requirements. Consulting with a registered dietitian or healthcare professional before making significant dietary changes is always recommended, especially if you have pre-existing health conditions. They can help you assess your individual needs, identify potential nutrient deficiencies, and develop a personalized plan that aligns with your health goals and overall well-being. This collaborative approach ensures a safe and effective transition to the Carnivore-Paleo way of eating.

The emphasis on individualization is crucial. The approach isn't about strict adherence to a rigid set of rules; it's about finding what works best for you. Experimentation within the framework of the philosophy is encouraged. You might find that incorporating certain vegetables, nuts, or seeds enhances your energy levels and overall well-being, while others may trigger discomfort or inflammation. This discovery process is vital for tailoring the diet to meet your unique needs and preferences, maximizing its benefits and supporting long-term sustainability. The goal isn't perfection, but progress—a steady, sustainable path toward improved health and well-being. Regular monitoring of your energy levels, sleep quality, and overall well-being helps guide adjustments and fine-tune the approach for optimal results.

Furthermore, the social aspects of eating should not be overlooked. Sharing meals with family and friends is a vital part of many cultures and promotes a sense of community. The Carnivore-Paleo approach does not necessarily preclude social gatherings; it's about making informed choices within social contexts. This may involve selecting restaurants with options that align with the dietary principles or preparing dishes that can be shared with others. It's about finding a balance that respects both your dietary preferences and your social connections. The key is mindful participation; being aware of your choices and enjoying the social aspect without compromising your dietary goals. Creative meal planning and communication with friends and family about your dietary choices can make it easier to enjoy social meals while maintaining your commitment to the Carnivore-Paleo philosophy.

Ultimately, the Carnivore-Paleo philosophy is more than just a diet; it's a holistic approach to health and well-being that emphasizes whole foods, mindful eating, and a long-term commitment to sustainable lifestyle changes. It offers a pathway to improved weight management, reduced inflammation, and enhanced overall health. However, like any dietary approach, individualization, regular monitoring, and open communication with healthcare professionals are crucial for optimal success and long-term adherence. The journey towards a healthier lifestyle is not a race, but a progressive process; embracing the holistic principles of this approach paves the way for lasting changes and improvements in your overall quality of life. By embracing the philosophy and adapting it to your individual needs and preferences, you embark on a path towards lasting well-being.

HighProtein HighFat Starts

Starting your day with a high-protein, high-fat breakfast is crucial for success on a Carnivore-Paleo approach. This isn't about deprivation; it's about fueling your body for optimal energy, satiety, and sustained weight management. Forget the sugary cereals and carb-laden pastries—we're focusing on nutrient-dense foods that will keep you full and energized until lunchtime.

One of the simplest and most satisfying breakfast options is a hearty serving of scrambled eggs. Eggs are nutritional powerhouses, packed with protein, healthy fats, and essential vitamins and minerals. A few variations can keep things exciting:

Classic Scrambled Eggs with Bacon:
This timeless
combination provides a perfect balance of protein and fat. Use high-quality bacon, ideally from pasture-raised pigs, for added flavor and nutritional benefits. Consider adding a sprinkle of sea salt and freshly ground black pepper for enhanced taste. The fat content in the bacon helps slow down the digestion of the eggs, promoting a longer-lasting feeling of fullness.

Scrambled Eggs with Avocado and Everything Bagel Seasoning:
For a creamier, more flavorful twist, add sliced avocado to your scrambled eggs. The healthy fats in avocado further enhance satiety and provide essential nutrients. A sprinkle of everything bagel seasoning adds a surprising burst of flavor. This option is particularly beneficial for those who miss the complexity of flavors found in less restrictive diets.

Keto Egg Bites:
Prepare a batch of keto egg bites ahead of time for a grab-and-go breakfast option. These can be
customized with various additions like sautéed mushrooms, cheese, or cooked bacon. The combination of egg protein and healthy fats ensures sustained energy levels throughout the morning. Ensure to use only healthy, low-carbohydrate cheese such as cheddar or mozzarella.

Beyond scrambled eggs, other excellent high-protein, high-fat breakfast options exist:

Bone Broth:
A warm cup of bone broth is a fantastic way to start the day, especially during colder months. It's rich in collagen, glycine, and other essential amino acids, promoting gut health and satiety. Bone broth can be enjoyed on its own or used as a base for other breakfast dishes, adding a savory depth to many meals. Consider adding a splash of apple cider vinegar for enhanced flavor and digestive benefits.

Fatty Cuts of Meat:
Don't underestimate the power of a simple serving of leftover steak or roast. These provide a substantial dose of protein and healthy fats, keeping you satisfied for hours. The ease and convenience of using leftovers also make it a good choice for those with busy schedules. Be mindful of the cooking method and seasoning to enhance the flavor and enjoyment.

Salmon with a Side of Avocado:
For a more elegant and nutrient-rich breakfast, consider smoked or cooked salmon with a side of avocado. Salmon is an excellent source of omega-3 fatty acids, protein, and essential vitamins. The avocado provides healthy fats and creamy texture,
complementing the flavor of the salmon perfectly.

Full-Fat Yogurt with Berries (Optional):
For those following a more liberal Carnivore-Paleo
approach that

incorporates some fruits, full-fat Greek yogurt with a small serving of berries (like blueberries or raspberries) can offer a refreshing and nutritious breakfast option. Choose plain, unsweetened yogurt and be mindful of the berry portion size to stay within carbohydrate targets. The fat in the yogurt will significantly improve satiety and ensure you are not left feeling hungry after your morning meal.

Nutritional Considerations and Recipe Examples:

Let's delve into the nutritional aspects and provide specific recipe examples for some of the breakfast options mentioned above:

Recipe 1: Classic Scrambled Eggs with Bacon (Serves 1)

Ingredients:
2 large eggs
2 slices of bacon (choose high-quality bacon)
Salt and freshly ground black pepper to taste

Instructions:
1. Cook bacon until crispy. Set aside on a paper towel-lined plate to drain excess fat.
2. Whisk eggs in a bowl with salt and pepper.
3. Cook eggs in a lightly oiled pan over medium heat, stirring occasionally, until cooked through.
4. Serve scrambled eggs with crispy bacon.

Nutritional Information (Approximate):
Calories: 350-400; Protein: 25-30g; Fat: 25-30g; Carbohydrates: <1g

Recipe 2: Scrambled Eggs with Avocado and Everything Bagel Seasoning (Serves 1)

Ingredients:

2 large eggs
½ avocado, sliced
Everything bagel seasoning to taste
Salt and pepper to taste

Instructions:
1. Whisk eggs with salt and pepper.
2. Cook eggs in a lightly oiled pan over medium heat, stirring occasionally, until cooked through.
3. Top with sliced avocado and everything bagel seasoning.

Nutritional Information (Approximate):
Calories: 300-350; Protein: 20-25g; Fat: 20-25g; Carbohydrates: 5-7g

Recipe 3: Keto Egg Bites (Makes 6 servings)

Ingredients:
6 large eggs
2 slices of bacon, cooked and crumbled½ cup shredded cheddar cheese
Salt and pepper to taste

Instructions:
1. Preheat oven to 300°F (150°C).
2. Grease a muffin tin.
3. Whisk eggs with salt and pepper.
4. Divide bacon and cheese evenly among muffin cups.
5. Pour egg mixture over bacon and cheese.
6. Bake for 20-25 minutes, or until set.

Nutritional Information (Approximate per serving):
Calories: 100-120; Protein: 7-8g; Fat: 8-10g; Carbohydrates: <1g

Recipe 4: Bone Broth (Serves 1)

Ingredients:
1 cup homemade or store-bought bone broth (ensure low-sodium options).
Optional: Pinch of sea salt, freshly ground black pepper, or a splash of apple cider vinegar for extra flavor.

Instructions:
Simply heat the bone broth gently until warm and enjoy.

Nutritional Information (Approximate):
Varies greatly depending on the ingredients and preparation. Protein is roughly 1-3g per cup.

Remember to adjust portion sizes based on your individual caloric needs and goals. These are just a few examples; feel free to experiment with different combinations of protein and fat sources to find what suits your palate and nutritional needs best. The key is consistency and choosing whole, unprocessed foods that align with the Carnivore-Paleo principles. Don't be afraid to get creative and personalize your breakfast to make it a delicious and enjoyable start to your day. The most important aspect is finding a breakfast routine that you can maintain easily and consistently, promoting long-term success in your weight loss journey.

Satisfying and Portable Meals

Lunchtime on a Carnivore-Paleo approach shouldn't be a source of stress. The goal is to continue the momentum established at breakfast, maintaining satiety and providing your body with the necessary nutrients to support your energy levels and weight loss goals. This means focusing on easily portable, high-protein, high-fat meals that are simple to prepare and enjoy, even on the go. Forget the complicated salads drowning in low-fat dressings or the sad desk lunch. We are building a lunch system that fuels your body and keeps you feeling satisfied until dinner.

Let's delve into the practicality of creating delicious and satisfying lunches that perfectly align with the Carnivore-Paleo principles. The key is to leverage leftovers from dinner, emphasizing preparation efficiency and minimizing mealtime stress. Think of your dinner as a two-for-one deal – one meal for tonight, and the other ready-to-go for tomorrow's lunch. This approach significantly reduces the burden of daily food preparation, making your weight-loss journey less demanding and more sustainable.

One of the simplest and most effective lunch strategies is repurposing dinner leftovers. If you roasted a chicken on Sunday, you have enough for several lunches during the week. Simply shred the leftover chicken and combine it with a generous helping of healthy fats, such as avocado or mayonnaise. This combination offers a satisfying and balanced meal, providing a significant protein source to sustain you throughout the afternoon. You can enjoy this on its own, or you can prepare simple salads featuring hearty greens, shredded chicken, and a drizzle of olive oil for a touch of additional healthy fats.

Let's explore some examples of how you can cleverly transform your dinners into satisfying and portable lunches. A hearty beef stew, rich in bone broth and tender beef, can be easily packed in a thermos and enjoyed hot, even hours later. The comforting warmth is a perfect antidote to a chilly afternoon, offering both nourishment and comfort. Leftover steak, grilled salmon, or pork chops can be equally easy to re-purpose. Simply slice or dice these proteins and pair them with some avocado slices, a dollop of sour cream or full-fat Greek yogurt, and you have yourself a satisfying and balanced meal.

For those who prefer salads, the Carnivore-Paleo approach offers a different perspective. Forget the low-fat, carb-loaded salads of the past. We are creating a powerhouse of nutrition. Instead, construct your salad around a base of hearty greens, adding generous portions of protein sources such as grilled chicken or beef, and finishing it with healthy fats. This might include avocado slices, olive oil, a sprinkle of macadamia nuts (if tolerated), or a dollop of full-fat mayonnaise. The key here is not to skimp on the healthy fats, as they contribute significantly to satiety and enhance the overall nutritional value of the meal. A small handful of olives would add a burst of flavour and healthy fats as well.

The beauty of this approach lies in its adaptability. If you prefer a more substantial salad, consider larger pieces of leftover roast beef or chicken. If you are on the go, a smaller salad with a protein-rich filling offers a convenient and satisfying option. Consider a simple combination such as leftover roast chicken breast combined with a small amount of shredded cheddar cheese and a dollop of full-fat mayonnaise.

For individuals who find themselves constantly on the move, portable lunch options are key to maintaining the Carnivore-Paleo approach throughout the day. One excellent choice is a hard-boiled egg, a significant source of protein and healthy fats. Pair this with a small container of full-fat cheese, such as cheddar or parmesan, for an extra protein and fat boost. The combination is both filling and easy to eat on the go. If you prefer something a little different, try a few slices of leftover cooked bacon – a delicious and convenient source of protein and saturated fat.

Another readily portable lunch option involves preparing a large batch of protein-rich meatballs in advance. These meatballs can be made with a blend of ground beef and pork, creating a dense and satisfying meal. You can simply pack a few meatballs in a container and enjoy them throughout the week. You could pack them with some cheese slices, or a small portion of full-fat yogurt for extra flavor and texture.

Let's not overlook the power of bone broth. A warm cup of bone broth is not only incredibly nutritious, but also incredibly satisfying. Its rich amino acid profile and gelatin content contribute to both satiety and gut health, making it a perfect lunch option for those seeking a lighter meal. You can enhance the flavor of your bone broth by adding a sprinkle of herbs or a dash of salt and pepper. Bone broth is extremely portable in a thermos and keeps you warm, especially during the colder months. It is also a very easy option to prepare on a busy day.

Consider a lunchbox that allows for separate compartments. This type of container enables you to portion your food effectively, ensuring you are consuming the right amount and keeping different food items separated, preserving freshness and texture. For instance, you can use a compartment for your protein (e.g., leftover steak or chicken), another for your healthy fats (e.g., avocado or a small amount of olive oil), and perhaps a small container for a side of cheese or olives. This compartmentalized approach encourages mindful eating and helps to manage portions more effectively.

Meal prepping on a weekend is another key to success. Prepare a large batch of hard-boiled eggs, roast a large quantity of chicken or beef, or make a big pot of bone broth. These pre-prepared elements significantly reduce the daily effort required for preparing lunch, making the entire process more manageable and less stressful, thus increasing adherence to the plan.

Beyond the specific recipes and suggestions, remember that flexibility and personalization are essential. The Carnivore-Paleo approach isn't about rigid adherence to a strict set of rules; it's about finding what works best for your individual needs and preferences. Experiment with different combinations of protein and fat sources to discover your favorite lunch options. The goal is to find a system that you can easily sustain long-term, which is significantly more important than achieving short-term weight loss results.

Listen to your body. Pay attention to how different foods make you feel. If you find that a particular combination leaves you feeling sluggish or unsatisfied, try something different. The process of discovering your optimal lunch routine is part of the overall journey. Don't be discouraged by initial experimentation; it is a normal part of the process.

Finally, remember the importance of hydration. Carry a water bottle with you throughout the day and aim to sip water regularly. Adequate hydration not only supports overall health but also aids in satiety, preventing you from mistaking thirst for hunger.

By focusing on simple, nutrient-dense meals, utilizing leftovers effectively, and embracing a flexible approach, you can easily create delicious and satisfying lunches that perfectly support your Carnivore-Paleo journey and help you achieve your weight loss goals. The key is consistency and finding a sustainable eating pattern that aligns with your lifestyle and preferences. Remember, this is a journey, not a race.

Flavorful and NutrientDense

Dinnertime is often considered the most challenging meal of the day, especially when adhering to a restrictive diet. However, with the Carnivore-Paleo approach, dinner can be a delightful and satisfying experience, far from the restrictive image often associated with weight loss diets. The key lies in embracing simplicity, utilizing high-quality ingredients, and focusing on nutrient density rather than calorie restriction. We are aiming for sustained satiety and the nourishment your body needs to recover and repair after a day of activity.

Let's explore some delicious and versatile dinner options that perfectly fit within the Carnivore-Paleo framework. We'll focus on recipes that are easy to prepare, requiring minimal cooking skills and readily available ingredients. Remember, the beauty of this approach lies in its adaptability; feel free to adjust the recipes according to your personal preferences and dietary needs. Always prioritize high-quality ingredients, sourced locally whenever possible.

Hearty Beef Stew:
A classic comfort food, reimagined for the Carnivore-Paleo lifestyle. This stew is rich in protein and healthy fats, providing sustained energy and keeping you full for hours.

Ingredients:
1.5 lbs beef stew meat, cut into 1-inch cubes; 1 large onion, roughly chopped; 2 carrots, roughly chopped; 2 celery stalks, roughly chopped; 4 cups beef broth (ensure it's low-sodium and free of added sugars); 2 tbsp bone marrow (optional, for extra richness and nutrients); 2 tbsp olive oil (or tallow); 1 tsp salt; 1/2 tsp black pepper; 1 bay leaf; 1 tsp dried thyme.

Instructions:
In a large pot or Dutch oven, heat the olive oil (or tallow) over medium-high heat. Brown the beef cubes in batches, ensuring not to overcrowd the pot. This step
enhances the flavor and texture. Remove the browned beef and set aside. Add the onion, carrots, and celery to the pot and cook until softened, about 5-7 minutes. Return the beef to the pot. Pour in the beef broth, add the bone marrow (if using), salt, pepper, bay leaf, and thyme. Bring the mixture to a boil, then reduce heat to low, cover, and simmer for at least 2-3 hours, or until the beef is incredibly tender. The longer it simmers, the more tender and flavorful the stew will become. Before serving, remove the bay leaf. This stew can be enjoyed on its own or served over a bed of cauliflower mash for added texture and nutrients.

Nutritional Information (per serving, approximate):
This will vary based on the specific ingredients and portion size.
However, a reasonable estimate would be around 400-500 calories, 40-50g of protein, and 25-35g of fat. The exact macronutrient breakdown can be calculated using a nutrition tracking app based on your specific ingredients and portion size.

Grilled Salmon with Asparagus:
A lighter yet equally satisfying dinner option, rich in omega-3 fatty acids and other essential nutrients.

Ingredients:
Two 6-ounce salmon fillets, skin on or off; 1 bunch asparagus, trimmed; 2 tbsp olive oil (or avocado oil); 1 tbsp lemon juice; salt and pepper to taste.

Instructions:
Preheat your grill to medium-high heat.
Lightly brush the salmon fillets and asparagus with olive oil. Season generously with salt and pepper. Place the salmon and asparagus on the grill. Cook the salmon for 4-6 minutes per side, or until cooked through. Cook the asparagus until

tender-crisp, about 5-7 minutes. Squeeze fresh lemon juice over the cooked salmon and asparagus before serving. This simple dish is packed with flavor and healthy fats, providing a perfect balance of nutrients.

Nutritional Information (per serving, approximate):
Around 400-450 calories, 30-35g of protein, and 25-30g of fat, with a significant amount of omega-3 fatty acids from the salmon. Again, the precise nutritional values depend on the specific ingredients and serving sizes.

Sheet Pan Chicken and Vegetables:
A convenient and flavorful option, perfect for busy weeknights. This recipe is highly adaptable; you can easily swap the vegetables
according to your preferences and seasonal availability.

Ingredients:
1.5 lbs boneless, skinless chicken thighs (or breasts); 1 lb broccoli florets; 1 red bell pepper, chopped; 1 yellow bell pepper, chopped; 2 tbsp olive oil; 1 tsp garlic powder; 1 tsp onion powder; salt and pepper to taste.

Instructions:
Preheat oven to 400°F (200°C). Toss the chicken and vegetables with olive oil, garlic powder, onion powder, salt, and pepper. Spread them in a single layer on a large baking sheet. Roast for 25-30 minutes, or until the chicken is cooked through and the vegetables are tender. This method minimizes cleanup and offers a balanced meal with protein and fiber.

Nutritional Information (per serving, approximate):
Around 450-550 calories, 40-50g of protein, and 20-25g of fat, with a good source of vitamins and minerals from the vegetables. Accurate values require specific ingredient and portion size data input into a nutrition tracker.

Bone Broth-Based Soup with Ground Beef:
This recipe emphasizes nutrient-rich bone broth, providing collagen and minerals essential for joint health and overall well-being.

Ingredients:
4 cups homemade bone broth (or high-quality store-bought bone broth); 1 lb ground beef; 1 onion, chopped; 2 carrots, chopped; 2 celery stalks, chopped; 1 tsp salt; 1/2 tsp black pepper; 1 bay leaf; fresh parsley (optional, for garnish).

Instructions:
In a large pot, brown the ground beef over medium heat. Add the onion, carrots, and celery and cook until softened, about 5-7 minutes. Pour in the bone broth, add the salt, pepper, and bay leaf. Bring the mixture to a boil, then reduce heat to low and simmer for at least 30 minutes, or until the vegetables are tender. Before serving, remove the bay leaf and garnish with fresh parsley if desired. This comforting soup is a powerhouse of nutrients, promoting gut health and overall well-being.

Nutritional Information (per serving, approximate):
Around 350-400 calories, 35-40g of protein, and 15-20g of fat. The nutritional content will change based on the specific ingredients and serving sizes.

Simple Pan-Seared Steak with Garlic Butter:
A quick and elegant dinner option that showcases the quality of the meat. Choose a high-quality cut of steak, such as ribeye, sirloin, or filet mignon.

Ingredients:
1 (8-ounce) steak; 2 tbsp butter; 2 cloves garlic, minced; salt and pepper to taste.

Instructions:
Season the steak generously with salt and pepper. Melt the

butter in a cast-iron skillet over medium-high heat. Add the minced garlic to the melted butter and cook for about 30 seconds, until fragrant. Sear the steak in the garlic butter for 3-4 minutes per side for medium-rare, or longer for your desired doneness. Let the steak rest for a few minutes before slicing and serving. This simple preparation highlights the natural flavor of the steak.

Nutritional Information (per serving, approximate): Around 400-500 calories, 40-50g of protein, and 30-35g of fat. The nutritional values vary widely depending on the type of steak and serving size.

These are just a few examples of the many delicious and nutrient-dense dinner options available within the Carnivore-Paleo framework. Remember to adjust the recipes to your taste preferences and dietary needs. The key is to focus on high-quality, whole foods and to prioritize simplicity in your meal preparation. Experiment with different spices and herbs to add variety and flavor to your meals. With a little creativity and planning, you can easily create delicious and satisfying dinners that support your weight loss goals and contribute to a healthier lifestyle. Remember to consult a healthcare professional or registered dietitian before making significant dietary changes, especially if you have any underlying health conditions. They can help you tailor a plan that meets your individual needs and preferences. Your journey to a healthier you begins with one delicious and nutritious meal at a time. Enjoy the process!

Maintaining Satiety Between Meals

The success of any weight-loss journey hinges not only on carefully planned meals but also on effectively managing those moments between meals – the times when hunger pangs can derail even the most determined efforts. The Carnivore-Paleo approach, with its emphasis on whole, nutrient-dense foods, offers unique advantages in combating those mid-day or evening cravings. The key lies in choosing snacks that promote satiety, keeping you feeling full and energized without disrupting your overall caloric balance or derailing your progress. Forget the processed, sugary snacks that lead to energy crashes and further cravings. We're focusing on real food, simple and satisfying.

One of the significant advantages of this dietary approach is the inherent satiety offered by the foods themselves. High-protein, high-fat foods naturally keep you feeling fuller for longer, reducing the urge to snack excessively. This isn't about deprivation; it's about strategic selection to maintain stable blood sugar levels and minimize hunger. Let's explore some effective snacking strategies.

Protein-Powered Snacks:
When choosing snacks, prioritize protein. Protein takes longer to digest than carbohydrates, leading to a prolonged feeling of fullness. A handful of hard-boiled eggs, for example, provides a substantial protein boost and keeps you satisfied until your next meal. Similarly, a small serving of leftover cooked meat (think steak,
chicken, or fish) offers a convenient and protein-rich snack option. The key is to prepare these in advance so you have them readily available when hunger strikes. Portion control is crucial here; even healthy, protein-rich snacks contribute to your overall calorie intake.

Healthy Fats: The Satiety Secret:
Don't underestimate the power of healthy fats in managing hunger. Fat is the most satiating macronutrient, meaning it keeps you feeling full for a longer period. A small portion of cheese, particularly
harder cheeses like cheddar or parmesan, provides a good dose of protein and fat, effectively combating cravings. A few slices of avocado, rich in monounsaturated fats, can also contribute to satiety and provide essential nutrients. Consider adding a small amount of healthy fat to your protein-based snacks; for example, a hard-boiled egg with a dollop of mayonnaise or a small piece of cheese with a few macadamia nuts can offer a satisfying combination of protein and fat.

Bone Broth's Unsung Benefits:
Bone broth, often
overlooked, is a fantastic snack option. Rich in collagen and other nutrients, it is incredibly satisfying and can be enjoyed warm or cold. It is easily digestible and provides a light yet filling snack, particularly beneficial if you experience afternoon sluggishness. Preparing a large batch on the weekend provides ample servings for the week ahead, ready for convenient snacking. Adding a dash of salt or some herbs and spices can enhance the flavor.

Beyond the Basics: Exploring Additional Options:

While the above options are excellent starting points, the Carnivore-Paleo approach allows for flexibility within its framework. Let's delve into some additional snacking strategies:

Leftovers:
Repurpose leftover dinner into satisfying snacks.
A few bites of roasted meat or vegetables can quell mid-afternoon hunger effectively. This minimizes food waste and maximizes convenience.

Nuts and Seeds (Optional and in Moderation):
While the Carnivore diet strictly adheres to animal products, some proponents of the Carnivore-Paleo approach occasionally include small portions of nuts and seeds, providing
additional healthy fats. Remember to exercise moderation due to the potential for high calorie density. Macadamia nuts, almonds, and Brazil nuts are good choices. Choose unsalted varieties to control sodium intake.

Olives:
These briny treats provide healthy fats and are naturally low in carbohydrates. They can be a satisfying snack, particularly when paired with a small amount of cheese.

Full-Fat Yogurt (Optional):
If dairy is tolerated, full-fat plain yogurt (without added sugars) can provide a good source of protein and fat. Be mindful of added sugars and choose unsweetened varieties.

Snack Timing and Portion Control:

The timing and portion size of your snacks are equally important. Avoid grazing throughout the day; instead, plan a couple of strategically timed snacks to maintain satiety without overconsuming calories. Pay attention to your hunger cues. A small snack might suffice if your hunger is mild, while a larger portion might be needed if you're feeling significantly hungry. Be mindful of your overall calorie intake; even healthy snacks contribute to your daily energy balance. Weigh and measure your snacks initially to help calibrate your portion sizes.

Hydration: The Often-Overlooked Factor:

Often mistaken for hunger, thirst can easily lead to unnecessary snacking. Ensure adequate hydration throughout the day. Carry a water bottle and sip consistently. Drinking water before a meal or snack can also help to reduce your overall food intake by creating a sense of fullness. Consider adding electrolytes to your water, particularly during periods of increased physical activity, to maintain hydration balance and prevent muscle cramps.

Listening to Your Body:

This is crucial. Pay attention to your body's signals. True hunger is different from emotional eating or boredom snacking. Before reaching for a snack, ask yourself if you're truly hungry or if you're simply bored or stressed. If you're not genuinely hungry, find another activity to distract yourself. Engage in a short walk, read a book, or call a friend; finding healthy distractions is vital to successful weight management.

Meal Timing and Snack Integration:

The timing of your meals also influences your snacking habits. Regular, well-spaced meals help to regulate blood sugar levels and reduce the likelihood of experiencing intense cravings between meals. If you tend to feel excessively hungry between meals, consider increasing your portion sizes at your main meals, ensuring you're consuming enough protein and fat to keep you satisfied for longer. This adjustment might reduce the need for additional snacks.

Addressing Potential Challenges:

While this approach emphasizes satiety, some individuals might still experience cravings or hunger. If you find yourself frequently hungry, consider several possibilities:

Macronutrient Ratios:
Are you consuming enough fat and protein? A lack of these essential macronutrients can lead to

increased hunger. Adjust your meal composition to include more protein and healthy fats.

Electrolyte Balance:
Electrolyte imbalances can sometimes mimic hunger. Ensure you're consuming adequate sodium, potassium, and magnesium through your food choices or supplementation (always under a healthcare professional's guidance).

Underlying Medical Conditions:
Certain medical
conditions can affect hunger and metabolism. Consult your doctor or a registered dietitian to rule out any underlying health issues.

Sleep Deprivation:
Lack of sleep significantly impacts hunger hormones, potentially increasing cravings. Prioritize getting adequate sleep to regulate appetite and enhance overall well-being.

Long-Term Sustainability:

The key to success with any dietary approach lies in its long-term sustainability. The Carnivore-Paleo principles, while offering a structured framework, should not feel restrictive. Experiment with different snack options and find what works best for you. This is a journey of discovery, and finding the right balance requires self-awareness and experimentation. Remember to listen to your body, adjust your plan as needed, and celebrate your progress along the way. Sustainable weight loss isn't a race; it's a marathon, and finding enjoyment in the process is crucial for long-term success. By focusing on whole, nutrient-dense foods and creating a satisfying eating pattern, you can pave the way for lasting weight management and improved overall health.

Making it Easy and Efficient

The cornerstone of successful weight loss, particularly with a Carnivore-Paleo approach, lies in consistent, well-planned meals. However, the perceived challenge of constantly preparing fresh meals can often deter individuals from embarking on, or sticking with, a new dietary regimen. This section aims to dispel that myth by providing practical, efficient, and time-saving meal preparation strategies that make adhering to a Carnivore-Paleo lifestyle both manageable and enjoyable. We'll explore techniques that simplify the process, reducing the time commitment while maximizing nutritional value.

One of the most effective strategies is
batch cooking
. This involves preparing larger portions of food at once, storing them appropriately, and then utilizing these pre-cooked
components throughout the week. Imagine a Sunday afternoon dedicated to cooking a large batch of roasted chicken, a substantial quantity of ground beef, or a sizable amount of salmon. This single cooking session can provide the foundation for numerous meals throughout the week. The roasted chicken can become the centerpiece for salads, soups, or simply enjoyed on its own. Ground beef can be incorporated into various dishes like stir-fries (with allowed vegetables), chili (using only allowed ingredients), or simply served as a base for a hearty bowl. Similarly, cooked salmon can be used in salads, or incorporated into omelets or frittatas. The possibilities are vast and limited only by your imagination and the allowed ingredients within your chosen Carnivore-Paleo parameters.

The key to successful batch cooking lies in organization and planning. Begin by reviewing your planned weekly meals.

Identify common ingredients and consolidate your shopping list accordingly. Once you've purchased your ingredients, dedicate a block of time to prepare larger quantities of these core components. Efficient use of oven space is paramount. For instance, you could roast a whole chicken alongside a tray of vegetables (if incorporating vegetables into your plan) and a sheet pan of hard-boiled eggs all at the same time. This multi-tasking approach significantly minimizes overall cooking time.

Proper storage is crucial to maintaining food quality and preventing spoilage. Invest in airtight containers – glass or high-quality plastic – to store your cooked components. Label each container clearly with the contents and date of preparation. Store cooked meats and other perishable items in the refrigerator promptly. For longer-term storage, freezing is an excellent option. Portion your meals into freezer-safe containers for grab-and-go convenience. Remember to allow ample time for food to cool completely before refrigerating or freezing to prevent bacterial growth.

Beyond batch cooking,
meal prepping
takes a slightly
different approach. Instead of preparing bulk ingredients, you assemble entire meals ahead of time. This method works particularly well for individuals with busy schedules, as it eliminates the need for cooking each meal individually during the week. Imagine preparing five individual containers, each containing a complete meal. One might include a generous portion of grilled steak, a side of steamed broccoli (if allowed), and a dollop of avocado (if allowed). Another could consist of leftover roasted chicken, a side salad with olive oil and salt, and a handful of macadamia nuts (if allowed). Another might feature a simple but satisfying combination of ground beef, sauteed spinach (if allowed) and a poached egg. This approach makes mealtimes convenient and stress-free throughout the busy week.

While batch cooking focuses on preparing individual components, meal prepping focuses on building complete, ready-to-eat meals. Both strategies offer significant time-saving advantages, and some people blend both methods to achieve optimal efficiency. The choice ultimately depends on individual preferences and schedules.

Efficient meal preparation also involves mastering **time-saving cooking techniques**. Utilizing a pressure cooker or Instant Pot can significantly reduce cooking times for meats and vegetables. A pressure cooker can tenderize tougher cuts of meat in a fraction of the time it would take in a conventional oven or on the stovetop. Similarly, a slow cooker can be used to prepare hearty stews and braised meats overnight, freeing up your time during the day. These appliances are particularly beneficial for busy individuals who want to adhere to a nutrient-rich diet without spending hours in the kitchen.

Another time-saving technique is to embrace **simplicity in your recipes**. Opt for recipes with minimal ingredients and straightforward preparation methods. Don't be afraid to keep things simple. A perfectly cooked steak seasoned with salt and pepper can be just as satisfying and nutritionally valuable as a more elaborate dish. The focus should always remain on quality ingredients prepared in a straightforward, healthy manner. Overly complicated recipes often lead to frustration and can be a barrier to long-term adherence to your chosen dietary plan.

Consider also the power of **one-pan or sheet pan cooking**. This technique allows you to cook multiple ingredients simultaneously on a single pan, minimizing cleanup and saving valuable time. For example, you could roast chicken and vegetables on one sheet pan, creating a complete meal with minimal effort. This approach also reduces the number of dishes you need to wash, a significant bonus for busy individuals.

Furthermore, embrace
pre-cut vegetables
(if incorporating vegetables) where permissible. Many supermarkets now offer pre-washed, pre-cut vegetables, saving considerable preparation time. This time-saving measure should only be employed if you can be certain of the quality and origin of these pre-cut options. Choose reputable brands and always wash them thoroughly before consumption, even if labeled as pre-washed.

Finally, don't underestimate the value of
planning your meals for the week
. This seemingly simple step is crucial for efficient meal preparation. A weekly meal plan serves as a roadmap, guiding your grocery shopping and ensuring you have all the necessary ingredients on hand. It eliminates impulsive decisions and the temptation to opt for less healthy options when you're tired or short on time. Having a clear plan minimizes waste and maximizes the utilization of ingredients, contributing to both cost savings and reduced food waste.

By incorporating these practical tips into your routine –batch cooking, meal prepping, utilizing time-saving cooking techniques, keeping recipes simple, embracing one-pan cooking, and employing pre-cut vegetables where appropriate - you can transform the often-daunting task of meal preparation into a manageable and efficient process. The focus should always be on creating a sustainable approach to dietary adherence that aligns with your lifestyle and preferences. Remember, successful weight loss is not about perfection; it's about consistently making healthy choices and employing strategies that work for you. By streamlining your meal preparation, you are investing in the success of your weight loss journey, laying the groundwork for lasting positive change.

The Importance of Water Intake

Water is often overlooked as a crucial component of weight loss and overall health, yet its role is paramount, particularly when following a Carnivore-Paleo approach. Adequate hydration isn't just about quenching thirst; it's fundamental to nearly every bodily function, impacting energy levels, metabolism, appetite regulation, and even the effectiveness of your diet. On a Carnivore-Paleo diet, where you're focusing on nutrient-dense, whole foods, ensuring proper hydration becomes even more critical.

Let's delve into why sufficient water intake is essential and explore practical strategies for staying properly hydrated throughout your day. Firstly, water plays a vital role in regulating body temperature. During physical activity, your body generates heat, and water helps dissipate this excess heat through sweating. Maintaining proper hydration is crucial to prevent overheating, particularly during intense workouts. On a Carnivore-Paleo diet, which often involves higher protein intake, adequate water intake becomes even more important due to the increased metabolic workload involved in protein digestion. Dehydration can lead to fatigue, decreased performance during workouts, and can even interfere with your body's ability to process nutrients effectively.

Secondly, water is crucial for optimal metabolic function. Many metabolic processes rely on water as a solvent and reactant. Your body uses water to break down food, transport nutrients to cells, and eliminate waste products. Dehydration can slow down these processes, making weight loss more challenging. Furthermore, adequate hydration helps to maintain optimal digestive function. Water helps soften stools, preventing constipation, which can be a common side effect of low-carbohydrate diets if hydration is neglected. Constipation can lead to discomfort, bloating, and can even hinder weight loss efforts.

Thirdly, water plays a significant role in appetite regulation. Many times, when we experience feelings of hunger, our bodies are actually signaling that they are dehydrated. Drinking water before a meal can help promote satiety and reduce overall caloric intake by filling the stomach and potentially reducing feelings of hunger. This is particularly useful when following a low-carbohydrate diet, as you are relying more on protein and fats to provide a sense of fullness. Many people mistakenly confuse thirst with hunger, leading to unnecessary snacking. By staying adequately hydrated, you can better differentiate between true hunger and thirst, preventing unnecessary calorie consumption.

Fourthly, water is essential for maintaining healthy skin. Adequate hydration keeps skin cells plump and hydrated, resulting in a healthier and more youthful appearance. The benefits extend beyond aesthetics; hydrated skin functions as a better barrier against environmental stressors, reducing inflammation and overall sensitivity. Given that many individuals experience improvements in skin conditions when following the Carnivore-Paleo diet, maintaining optimal hydration becomes even more important to support this beneficial effect.

Now, let's discuss practical strategies to ensure adequate hydration throughout the day. Start by keeping a water bottle with you at all times. This serves as a constant visual reminder to sip water regularly. Aim for consistent hydration throughout the day rather than trying to drink large amounts of water in sporadic intervals. A common strategy is to drink a glass of water before each meal. This helps to promote satiety, as previously mentioned, and sets a consistent hydration habit.

Consider adding some electrolytes to your water, particularly if you are engaging in strenuous physical activity. Electrolytes are essential minerals, such as sodium, potassium, and magnesium, that help regulate fluid balance and support muscle function. Electrolyte imbalances can lead to dehydration, muscle cramps, and fatigue. While natural electrolytes are found in many foods, adding an electrolyte supplement, especially during or after intense workouts, can be beneficial to prevent dehydration and electrolyte depletion. You can also boost your electrolyte intake through natural sources such as bone broth, which is a staple in the Carnivore-Paleo diet.

Monitor your urine color. A pale yellow or clear urine indicates adequate hydration. Darker yellow urine signals that you need to increase your water intake. This is a simple and effective way to assess your hydration status. Be mindful of the timing of your water consumption. Drinking a significant amount of water immediately before or during meals can sometimes dilute stomach acid, potentially affecting digestion. Space out your water intake evenly throughout the day for optimal hydration and digestive function.

For those who find it challenging to drink plain water, consider adding slices of lemon, lime, or cucumber to your water for a refreshing flavor. This adds a subtle taste without adding any significant calories or disrupting your dietary approach. Infused water is a popular strategy for those who struggle to consume enough plain water. Experiment with different combinations of fruits and vegetables to find a flavor that you enjoy. Remember, the goal is to make hydration a pleasant and enjoyable part of your daily routine.

Another crucial aspect to consider is the timing of your water intake. Consuming a large amount of water right before bed can lead to nighttime bathroom trips, disrupting your sleep. While maintaining adequate hydration is essential, it's wise to moderate your water intake closer to bedtime to avoid sleep disruptions. Listen to your body's signals, adjusting your water intake according to your activity level, climate, and individual needs. What works for one person may not work for another. Pay attention to how your body responds and adjust your hydration strategy accordingly.

In summary, adequate hydration is a cornerstone of successful weight loss and overall health, especially when following a Carnivore-Paleo approach. Prioritize consistent hydration throughout the day, incorporating strategies like keeping a water bottle handy, monitoring urine color, and adding flavorful additions to make it more enjoyable. Remember that hydration is not a one-size-fits-all approach. Experiment to find a strategy that works best for you and allows you to comfortably maintain optimal hydration levels for long-term success. Remember to consult with your healthcare provider or a registered dietitian if you have any concerns regarding your hydration status or dietary plan. They can help you create a personalized hydration strategy that aligns with your individual needs and health goals. By prioritizing hydration, you're investing in your overall well-being and enhancing the effectiveness of your Carnivore-Paleo journey.

Monitoring Your Weight and Measurements

Progress tracking is an essential element of any successful weight loss journey, and the Carnivore-Paleo approach is no exception. However, it's crucial to approach this aspect with a balanced perspective. While numbers provide valuable insights, they shouldn't become the sole focus, leading to obsession or discouragement. The goal is to use data to inform your journey, not define your worth.

Begin by selecting a consistent method for measuring your progress. This might involve weighing yourself weekly, using a body composition scale to monitor fat mass and muscle mass, or employing a combination of methods. The most effective strategy will depend on your individual preferences and goals. If you're using a scale, weigh yourself at the same time of day, ideally in the morning before eating or drinking, to minimize daily fluctuations. Wearing similar clothing each time will also help ensure accuracy.

Body composition scales, often found at gyms or pharmacies, provide a more comprehensive picture of your body composition, going beyond just weight to measure things like body fat percentage, muscle mass, and water retention. This information can be particularly helpful in monitoring progress when weight loss plateaus, as it allows you to see if you're losing fat while gaining muscle, even if the overall weight change isn't significant.

Beyond weight and body composition, consider tracking other measurements, such as waist circumference, hip circumference, or other body measurements you find relevant. These measurements can be particularly useful in identifying changes in specific areas of your body, providing a more detailed picture of your progress. Take these measurements at the same time of day, using a tape measure, ensuring it's held snugly but not too tightly.

Photography can be a powerful tool for progress tracking. Taking photos weekly or bi-weekly allows you to visually observe your changes, providing a less numerical, more holistic perspective. Remember to take consistent photos from the same angle and in the same lighting conditions to ensure accurate comparison.

While numbers are valuable, remember that they represent only one aspect of your progress. Focus on non-scale victories, such as improvements in your energy levels, sleep quality, digestion, and overall mood. Note these positive changes in a journal or tracking app, celebrating every small step forward. This broader perspective prevents you from solely focusing on the numbers on the scale, which can be disheartening if weight loss slows down temporarily.

Consistent monitoring is essential, but avoid obsessive weighing or measuring. Daily weigh-ins can lead to unnecessary stress and anxiety, as weight fluctuates naturally due to factors like fluid retention, hormonal changes, and food consumption. Aim for a weekly or bi-weekly schedule instead, allowing for a more accurate representation of your long-term progress.

It's crucial to be patient and persistent, recognizing that weight loss is not always linear. There will be weeks where the scale shows little or no change, or even a slight increase. These fluctuations are normal and don't indicate failure. Focus on the overall trend over several weeks or months, rather than getting discouraged by short-term fluctuations.

Furthermore, consider recording your food intake and physical activity levels. While not essential for everyone, this practice can provide valuable insights into your eating habits and identify areas for improvement. Using a food diary or app can help you track your calorie intake, macronutrient ratios, and identify patterns in your eating behavior. Similarly, tracking your physical activity can help you stay accountable and identify areas where you might increase your activity levels.

Remember that progress tracking is not about perfection; it's about awareness and self-understanding. The data you collect should empower you to make informed decisions about your diet and lifestyle, fostering a sustainable and healthy relationship with food and your body.

Let's delve deeper into some practical tips for effective progress tracking. Consistency is key. Choose a method—whether it's weighing, measuring, taking photos, or a combination—and stick to it. Having a consistent routine minimizes inconsistencies and makes it easier to track your progress over time. Select days and times that fit seamlessly into your schedule, so that tracking becomes a natural part of your routine.

Use a tracking method that works for you. If weighing yourself daily creates undue stress, opt for a less frequent approach. If you find numerical data overwhelming, prioritize photos or journaling about your non-scale victories. The aim is to find a system that motivates you, not demotivates you.

Embrace the process. Remember that progress isn't always linear, and setbacks are inevitable. Don't let a temporary plateau or a week of no significant weight loss derail your efforts. Focus on the long-term goals, celebrating small wins along the way.

Be honest with yourself. Accurate tracking requires honesty. Don't underreport your food intake or overestimate your physical activity. Accurate data is essential for making informed decisions about your diet and lifestyle choices.

Seek support when needed. If you're struggling to track your progress or feeling overwhelmed by the process, consider seeking support from a registered dietitian, a personal trainer, or a support group. They can offer guidance, accountability, and encouragement.

Beyond weight and measurements, consider incorporating other indicators of well-being into your tracking. This could include monitoring energy levels, sleep quality, mood, digestion, and pain levels. These aspects can provide a more holistic view of your progress and reveal potential areas for improvement. A journal can be a valuable tool for recording these qualitative changes.

Consider using technology to help you track your progress. There are many apps available that can help you track your weight, body measurements, food intake, and physical activity. These apps can provide valuable insights into your progress and help you stay motivated. Explore various apps to find one that meets your specific needs and preferences.

Finally, remember that the numbers are not the end-all, be-all. Focus on how you feel, your energy levels, and how well you're meeting your personal goals. If your measurements remain largely unchanged but you are experiencing significant improvements in your health and well-being, celebrate these achievements. The ultimate measure of success is a healthier, happier, and more energetic you. Use your progress tracking methods as tools for self-awareness and motivation, not as sources of judgment or self-criticism. Your journey is unique, and your progress should be celebrated in its own way. By integrating a comprehensive and balanced approach to progress tracking, you'll empower yourself to achieve sustainable weight loss and a healthier lifestyle on your Carnivore-Paleo journey.

Overcoming Challenges and Plateaus

Overcoming challenges is an inevitable part of any significant lifestyle change, and embarking on a Carnivore-Paleo journey is no exception. While the simplicity of this approach can be incredibly empowering, you may still encounter moments of doubt, frustration, or even setbacks. Understanding these potential hurdles and developing effective coping strategies is crucial for long-term success.

One common challenge is managing cravings. The initial transition away from processed foods, sugary drinks, and refined carbohydrates can trigger intense cravings, especially if you've been accustomed to a diet rich in these items. These cravings are often not about hunger but rather about learned associations and emotional responses to certain foods. To combat these cravings, focus on understanding their root causes. Are you bored? Stressed? Do you associate certain foods with particular emotions or social situations? Identifying these triggers is the first step towards managing them.

Instead of succumbing to cravings, consider strategies to address the underlying need. If stress is the culprit, try incorporating stress-reducing activities like yoga, meditation, or spending time in nature. If boredom is the issue, engage in a hobby or activity you enjoy. Remember that cravings are temporary; they typically subside after a few days or weeks as your body adjusts to its new nutritional state. To further reduce cravings, ensure you're consuming adequate protein and healthy fats to keep you feeling satiated. A well-planned Carnivore-Paleo meal plan will provide the essential nutrients needed to minimize these cravings. If cravings persist despite these strategies, consider consulting a registered dietitian or nutritionist specializing in low-carbohydrate diets for personalized guidance. They can help you identify any nutritional deficiencies that may be contributing to your cravings and develop strategies to address them.

Another significant hurdle is weight loss plateaus. These periods of stalled progress are common, and it's important not to become discouraged. Plateaus often occur due to several factors, including hormonal fluctuations, metabolic adaptation, and even inaccurate tracking. Your body is incredibly efficient at adapting to changes, and as you lose weight, your metabolism may slow down slightly. This doesn't mean your efforts are fruitless; it simply means your body requires adjustments to continue its progress.

When encountering a plateau, first meticulously review your tracking methods. Are you accurately measuring and logging your food intake? Are you consistently monitoring your physical activity? Minor inaccuracies can accumulate and obscure your progress. If your tracking is accurate, consider making minor adjustments to your diet or exercise routine. You can slightly increase your protein intake, introduce a new type of exercise, or vary your workout intensity. These adjustments can help to stimulate your metabolism and break through the plateau. Remember to make these changes gradually, allowing your body time to adjust. Sudden, drastic changes are more likely to lead to setbacks.

It's also essential to remember the importance of non-scale victories. Even when the scale doesn't reflect noticeable changes, you may be experiencing other positive improvements, such as increased energy levels, better sleep, improved mood, or reduced inflammation. Focus on these positive changes as evidence of your progress. Celebrate these non-scale victories as much as you celebrate weight loss milestones. These successes will reinforce your commitment and motivation to continue on your Carnivore-Paleo journey.

Another common obstacle is social situations. Maintaining a Carnivore-Paleo diet can present challenges when dining out or attending social gatherings where food choices may be limited. Don't be afraid to explain your dietary choices to your friends and family; most people are understanding and willing to accommodate your needs. However, be prepared to politely decline offerings that don't align with your dietary plan. You can choose to bring your own food, select dishes that are compatible with your diet, or simply focus on the social aspect of the gathering rather than the food. The key is to prioritize your health and wellness goals without being overly rigid or isolating yourself socially.

Planning ahead is crucial for success. Prepare meals in advance, especially for busy days or social events. This way, you'll always have healthy options available. When dining out, research restaurants in advance to identify establishments with options suitable for your dietary plan. This proactive approach will help you avoid impulsive choices and maintain consistency in your healthy eating habits. Remember, choosing healthy options isn't about deprivation; it's about making informed choices that align with your wellness goals.

Consistency is perhaps the most crucial factor in achieving long-term success. Remember that weight loss is a journey, not a race. There will be ups and downs, successes and setbacks. The key is not to let setbacks derail your progress. Instead, view them as learning opportunities and readjust your approach as needed. Consistency in your diet, exercise, and other healthy habits will ultimately determine your success.

Consider maintaining a journal to track your progress, reflect on your successes and challenges, and identify potential adjustments. This journal can be a valuable tool for self-reflection and motivation. It's also beneficial to seek support from others who are embarking on similar dietary changes. Sharing experiences and challenges with others who understand can provide invaluable encouragement and accountability. Consider online forums, support groups, or even just connecting with friends or family members who are supportive of your goals.

Electrolyte imbalances can also pose a challenge, particularly during the initial phases of the Carnivore-Paleo diet. As your body adapts to a lower carbohydrate intake, your electrolyte levels may fluctuate. Therefore, it's crucial to monitor and maintain appropriate levels of sodium, potassium, and magnesium. Adding salt to your meals, consuming electrolyte-rich broths, or using electrolyte supplements (if needed and under the guidance of a healthcare professional) can help prevent electrolyte imbalances and address related symptoms such as muscle cramps or fatigue. Listen to your body and adjust your electrolyte intake as needed.

Sleep deprivation can significantly hinder weight loss efforts. When you're sleep-deprived, your body produces more cortisol, a stress hormone that can promote fat storage. Prioritizing quality sleep (7-9 hours per night) is crucial for maintaining energy levels, managing stress, and supporting overall health and weight management goals. Establish a consistent sleep schedule, create a relaxing bedtime routine, and optimize your sleep environment for maximum restorative sleep.

Finally, remember that this journey is deeply personal. There's no one-size-fits-all approach to the Carnivore-Paleo diet. What works for one person may not work for another. Be patient, persistent, and flexible in your approach. Experiment with different meal plans, exercise routines, and strategies to discover what works best for you and your individual needs and preferences. Remember to celebrate every step of the way and focus on long-term lifestyle changes rather than quick fixes. This journey is about nourishing your body and improving your well-being, not just about losing weight. By focusing on sustainable habits and a holistic approach to wellness, you can achieve your weight loss goals and cultivate a healthier and happier life.

Managing Social Situations and Eating Out

Navigating social situations and eating out can present unique challenges when following the Carnivore-Paleo approach. The abundance of carbohydrate-laden options and the social pressure to conform can make sticking to your dietary plan feel overwhelming. However, with a little planning and a confident approach, you can easily enjoy social gatherings and dining out without compromising your health goals. The key is to remember that you're not depriving yourself; you're making conscious choices that benefit your well-being.

Preparation is paramount. Before attending any social event, mentally prepare yourself. Visualize scenarios where you might face temptation and anticipate how you'll respond. This proactive mental rehearsal can significantly reduce impulsive choices. Consider informing your host or close friends about your dietary preferences beforehand. A well-informed host is much more likely to accommodate your needs, perhaps even offering suitable options. Don't feel obligated to explain the specifics of your diet to everyone; a simple "I'm following a specific eating plan" is usually sufficient.

When attending parties or gatherings where food is served buffet-style, carefully survey the options before selecting your meal. Look for meat-centric choices such as grilled chicken, fish, or steak. Avoid processed meats laden with additives and fillers. Prioritize plain meat and vegetables if available; you can always add healthy fats like olive oil or avocado if desired. If there's nothing suitable, don't be afraid to bring your own dish! A simple salad with grilled chicken or a platter of hard-boiled eggs can be a satisfying and appropriate contribution.

Eating out at restaurants requires a more strategic approach. Research restaurants beforehand. Many establishments now cater to various dietary needs, including low-carb and Paleo options. Check their menus online to identify potential dishes that align with your plan. Look for restaurants specializing in steak, seafood, or grilled meats. When ordering, don't be afraid to ask for modifications. Request sides of steamed vegetables instead of starchy carbs. You can often substitute sauces or dressings for healthier alternatives. Be clear and assertive when requesting modifications; most restaurants are happy to accommodate reasonable requests.

Remember that portion control is crucial, even when eating out. The portions served in restaurants are often larger than necessary. Don't feel pressured to finish everything on your plate. Order a smaller portion or share a dish with a companion. If you find yourself facing a large portion, don't hesitate to take some home for another meal.

Dealing with unexpected situations requires adaptability and self-compassion. There will be occasions where finding completely compliant meal options is impossible. In such cases, prioritize your well-being. Focus on selecting the most suitable option available, even if it's not perfectly aligned with your Carnivore-Paleo approach. A minor deviation from your plan doesn't mean failure. It's about long-term consistency, not perfection. Remember to get back on track with your next meal. Don't let a single deviation derail your progress.

Social pressure is another common hurdle. Many people may express skepticism or even disapproval regarding your dietary choices. Remember that your health is your priority, and you have the right to choose what's best for your body. Be polite but firm in your responses. You don't need to justify your dietary decisions to anyone. If someone is persistently critical, gently redirect the conversation or politely excuse yourself. Your commitment to your well-being should not be undermined by the opinions of others.

Alcohol consumption can also be a challenge on a Carnivore-Paleo diet. Many alcoholic beverages are high in carbohydrates and sugars. If you choose to drink alcohol, opt for lower-carbohydrate options like dry red wine or spirits mixed with unsweetened seltzers or club soda. Always be mindful of your alcohol consumption, as it can interfere with your weight loss efforts and overall health. Remember, moderation is key.

Another crucial aspect is managing emotional eating. Social situations can often trigger emotional eating, even when following a strict diet. Identify your emotional triggers and develop coping mechanisms. Practice mindfulness and pay attention to your hunger cues. Distinguish between true hunger and emotional cravings. If you find yourself emotionally driven to eat, engage in alternative activities like taking a walk, calling a friend, or listening to music to distract yourself.

The role of mindful eating cannot be overstated, especially in social contexts. Slow down, savor each bite, and pay attention to the flavors and textures of your food. This mindful approach can help you feel more satisfied with smaller portions and reduce the likelihood of overeating. Avoid distractions like your phone or television while eating, allowing yourself to fully appreciate your meal.

Preparation extends beyond just food. Plan your outfits and activities to ensure you feel confident and comfortable. If possible, choose activities that don't revolve solely around food. Engage in conversations, play games, or participate in other activities that keep you occupied and distract you from focusing solely on food. This proactive approach can significantly reduce food-related stress.

Maintaining a supportive network is crucial. Surround yourself with people who understand and support your dietary goals. Sharing your journey with like-minded individuals can provide encouragement and accountability. Consider joining online support groups or connecting with others who follow similar dietary approaches. These supportive communities can provide invaluable resources and motivation.

Remember, success with the Carnivore-Paleo diet isn't just about weight loss; it's about a lifestyle change. It's about developing healthy habits and integrating them into your everyday life. Social situations should not feel like insurmountable obstacles; they should be opportunities to apply the skills and knowledge you've learned. By practicing these strategies, you can confidently navigate social settings and maintain a healthy and balanced approach to the Carnivore-Paleo lifestyle. It's about making conscious and informed decisions that support your long-term well-being. Enjoy the journey, be patient with yourself, and celebrate your successes along the way. The rewards of a healthier lifestyle extend far beyond weight loss – they encompass increased energy, improved mental clarity, and a greater sense of well-being. Remember that this lifestyle isn't a short-term fix; it's a sustainable path towards a healthier and happier you. Focus on building a foundation of healthy habits that you can maintain for years to come. Your health journey is a marathon, not a sprint. Celebrate small victories, learn from setbacks, and never give up on your commitment to a better you.

Building Sustainable Habits for LongTerm Success

The journey towards a healthier lifestyle, particularly when adopting a dietary approach like Carnivore-Paleo, is a marathon, not a sprint. Initial enthusiasm often fades if we don't build sustainable habits that seamlessly integrate into our daily routines. This is where the real work begins – establishing practices that support long-term adherence and prevent the inevitable plateaus and challenges that accompany any significant lifestyle change. The key is to shift from a mindset of restrictive dieting to one of mindful living, focusing on nourishing your body and mind consistently.

One of the most effective strategies for building sustainable habits is to start small. Don't try to overhaul your entire life overnight. Instead, focus on incorporating one or two new habits each week. For example, you might begin by preparing one Carnivore-Paleo meal a day, gradually increasing this until all your meals align with the plan. This approach prevents feeling overwhelmed and increases your chances of success. It's about gradual integration, not immediate transformation. Celebrate every small victory; the consistency of these small wins builds momentum and confidence.

Another powerful technique is habit stacking. This involves linking a new habit to an existing one. For example, if you already have a morning routine of brushing your teeth, you might add a habit of drinking a large glass of water immediately after. Or, if you always have your coffee before work, you could add preparing a simple Carnivore breakfast simultaneously. By associating the new habit with an established one, you create a natural trigger that increases the likelihood of consistent behavior. This seemingly small technique can significantly impact long-term adherence. The power of habit stacking lies in its simplicity and effectiveness in creating automated routines.

Meal prepping is a cornerstone of long-term success on any dietary plan, but particularly so with the Carnivore-Paleo approach. Setting aside a few hours each week to prepare meals and snacks in advance eliminates the temptation to grab unhealthy options when time is short. Batch cooking simple, versatile meals like bone broth, roasted meats, or hard-boiled eggs provides a readily available source of nutritious food, reducing the likelihood of impulsive, less healthy choices. This strategic preparation significantly reduces stress and eliminates decision fatigue, especially crucial during busy days. Consider portioning your prepped meals into individual containers for easy grab-and-go options throughout the week.

Mindful eating is another crucial component of building sustainable habits. This involves paying close attention to your body's hunger and fullness cues, savoring your food, and eating without distractions. Put away your phone, turn off the TV, and focus on the taste, texture, and aroma of your meal. This conscious engagement with your food enhances satisfaction and reduces the likelihood of overeating. Mindful eating also encourages better digestion and creates a more positive relationship with food. Regularly check in with yourself – are you truly hungry, or are you eating out of boredom, stress, or emotional triggers? Understanding your hunger cues is a critical step toward long-term success.

Hydration plays a surprisingly significant role in weight management and overall health. Drinking plenty of water throughout the day helps regulate your appetite, boost your metabolism, and improve digestion. Aim for at least eight glasses of water a day, and more if you are physically active. Consider carrying a reusable water bottle with you, making it readily available throughout your day. Infuse your water with slices of lemon or cucumber for a refreshing twist, if desired. The consistent intake of water supports numerous bodily functions, aiding in your overall health goals.

Tracking your progress, though seemingly trivial, provides invaluable insight and motivation. Monitoring your weight, body measurements, and energy levels helps you stay accountable and identify areas for improvement. Consider using a journal or a smartphone app to record your food intake, exercise, and overall well-being. Visualizing your progress can be highly motivating, highlighting achievements and guiding adjustments to your plan. However, remember to focus on non-scale victories too – improvements in sleep quality, energy levels, and mental clarity should also be celebrated. Don't solely rely on the number on the scale; the holistic picture is more revealing.

Prioritizing sleep is often overlooked but is paramount for success. Adequate sleep regulates hormones that control appetite and metabolism, making weight management more manageable. Aim for seven to nine hours of quality sleep each night. Establish a relaxing bedtime routine to help you unwind before sleep. This could include taking a warm bath, reading a book, or listening to calming music. A consistently restful sleep pattern is integral to a successful, long-term health transformation. The impact of sleep deprivation on hormonal balance cannot be understated in this context.

Incorporating regular physical activity into your routine is crucial for overall health and weight management. Choose activities you genuinely enjoy, whether it's walking, hiking, swimming, strength training, or HIIT workouts. Find an activity that fits your lifestyle and fitness level. Aim for at least 30 minutes of moderate-intensity exercise most days of the week. The key is consistency, not intensity; making physical activity a regular part of your life is far more impactful than sporadic bursts of high-intensity exercise. Look for opportunities to integrate more movement into your daily life; take the stairs instead of the elevator, park further away from your destination, or incorporate short walks during your workday.

Stress management is another important aspect of long-term success. Chronic stress can lead to overeating and hinder your progress. Find healthy ways to manage stress, such as meditation, yoga, spending time in nature, or engaging in hobbies you enjoy. Stress reduction techniques are not luxuries, but rather essential tools for sustainable health changes. Regularly incorporating stress-reducing activities is equally as important as regular exercise and healthy eating.

Seeking support from others can significantly improve adherence to your dietary plan. Connect with others following a similar lifestyle, either online or in person. Share experiences, challenges, and successes with your support system. A strong support network can boost motivation and provide valuable encouragement, especially during challenging periods. The communal aspect of shared goals fosters resilience and combats feelings of isolation which are common hurdles in adopting major lifestyle changes. Finding your tribe, whether online or offline, is invaluable.

Building sustainable habits requires patience, persistence, and self-compassion. There will be days when you stumble, and that's perfectly okay. Don't let setbacks derail your progress; instead, learn from them and move on. Celebrate your successes, no matter how small, and remember that progress is more important than perfection. The journey towards a healthier lifestyle is a continuous process of learning, adapting, and refining. Self-compassion is essential in navigating this journey, enabling consistent progress without overwhelming self-criticism.

Finally, remember that this lifestyle change isn't about deprivation; it's about nourishing your body with nutrient-dense foods and making choices that support your overall well-being. Enjoy the process, focus on the positive changes you're experiencing, and celebrate your successes along the way. The rewards of a healthier lifestyle extend far beyond weight loss; they encompass increased energy, improved mental clarity, a greater sense of well-being, and a significantly improved quality of life. Embrace the journey, and enjoy the transformation! Your commitment to a healthier you is an investment in a richer and more fulfilling life. This is not a diet; it's a lifestyle.

The Importance of Physical Activity for Weight Loss

Exercise isn't just about burning calories; it's a cornerstone of a holistic approach to weight loss and overall well-being. While dietary changes form the foundation of weight management on the Carnivore-Paleo approach, incorporating regular physical activity significantly amplifies its effectiveness. Think of it like this: diet provides the fuel efficiency of your car, while exercise is the accelerator, propelling you towards your weight-loss goals faster and more sustainably. Ignoring exercise is like only focusing on fuel efficiency—you might make progress, but it'll be slow and less impactful.

The benefits of exercise extend far beyond the scale. It boosts your metabolism, helping your body burn more calories even at rest. This metabolic boost is particularly crucial for long-term weight maintenance, as it prevents your body from slowing its metabolism in response to caloric restriction, a common problem with restrictive diets. Furthermore, exercise helps build and maintain lean muscle mass. Muscle tissue is metabolically active, meaning it burns more calories than fat tissue, even while you're resting. This increased muscle mass contributes to a higher resting metabolic rate, making it easier to maintain a healthy weight even after reaching your target.

Beyond the metabolic advantages, exercise plays a critical role in improving cardiovascular health, reducing the risk of chronic diseases like heart disease, stroke, and type 2 diabetes. These conditions are often associated with obesity and contribute to a host of other health problems. Regular physical activity strengthens your heart and improves its efficiency in pumping blood throughout your body. It also helps lower blood pressure and cholesterol levels, crucial factors in maintaining cardiovascular health.

Furthermore, the psychological benefits of exercise are invaluable for successful weight loss. Exercise combats stress, improves mood, and boosts self-esteem – all of which are critical in maintaining motivation and adherence to your diet and exercise plan. The endorphins released during exercise act as natural mood elevators, helping you combat the emotional eating often associated with stress and low self-esteem. The sense of accomplishment you feel after a workout further reinforces positive habits and builds confidence in your ability to achieve your weight-loss goals. This positive feedback loop contributes significantly to long-term success, making exercise not just a means to an end, but an integral part of a fulfilling and healthier lifestyle.

Choosing the right type of exercise is crucial. It's essential to select activities you genuinely enjoy, ensuring long-term adherence to your exercise plan. Avoid starting with rigorous and intense workouts if you're a beginner. Instead, opt for activities that are enjoyable and sustainable. Walking is a simple and highly accessible form of exercise, perfect for beginners. It's low-impact, easy on your joints, and can be incorporated into your daily routine without requiring specialized equipment or gym memberships. Start with shorter walks and gradually increase the duration and intensity as your fitness level improves. This gradual approach prevents burnout and injuries, ensuring you can continue exercising consistently.

Strength training is another essential component of a well-rounded exercise program. It's not just for bodybuilders; strength training is crucial for building lean muscle mass, improving bone density, and increasing your metabolic rate.

You don't need to lift heavy weights; bodyweight exercises like squats, push-ups, and lunges are excellent starting points. As you gain strength and confidence, you can incorporate resistance bands or light weights into your routine. Remember to focus on proper form to avoid injuries and maximize results. Consult a qualified fitness professional for guidance on proper form and exercise selection, particularly if you're new to strength training.

High-Intensity Interval Training (HIIT) is another effective way to boost your metabolism and burn calories in a short amount of time. HIIT involves short bursts of intense exercise followed by brief recovery periods. This type of training is very efficient, making it ideal for individuals with busy schedules. Examples of HIIT exercises include sprinting intervals, cycling intervals, or even bodyweight exercises like burpees and jumping jacks. Remember to listen to your body and adjust the intensity and duration of your HIIT workouts to avoid overexertion, especially when starting.

Finding a balance between these various exercise types is key. A balanced approach encompassing cardiovascular exercise (like walking or HIIT), strength training, and flexibility exercises (like yoga or stretching) ensures you work all major muscle groups, improve your cardiovascular health, and increase your flexibility and range of motion. This holistic approach promotes overall fitness and reduces your risk of injury.

Creating a sustainable exercise plan requires careful consideration of your individual circumstances. Start small and gradually increase the intensity and duration of your workouts. If you're starting with a sedentary lifestyle, aim for at least 30 minutes of moderate-intensity exercise most days of the week. This can be broken down into shorter sessions throughout the day to fit into your schedule. Be realistic and flexible; life happens, and it's okay to miss a workout occasionally. The key is to establish a consistent pattern rather than striving for perfection.

The integration of exercise with your Carnivore-Paleo diet is essential for maximizing weight loss results. Remember that exercise enhances the effects of caloric restriction by boosting your metabolism and increasing your energy expenditure. By combining a nutrient-dense diet with regular exercise, you create a synergistic effect that propels your weight loss journey and significantly improves your overall health and fitness levels.

Listening to your body is crucial throughout your exercise journey. Pay attention to signals of fatigue, pain, or discomfort. Rest and recovery are just as important as exercise itself. Overtraining can lead to injuries, burnout, and hinder your progress. Allow for rest days to allow your body to repair and rebuild muscle tissue. Adequate sleep also plays a significant role in recovery and maximizing your exercise benefits. Prioritize sleep to optimize your energy levels and enhance the positive effects of your workout routine.

Avoid comparing your progress to others; everyone's journey is unique. Focus on your own personal progress and celebrate small victories along the way. Remember that weight loss is a journey, not a race. Be patient, persistent, and kind to yourself throughout the process. Incorporating physical activity is not merely a component of weight loss; it's a fundamental element of a healthier and more fulfilling lifestyle. The combination of a well-planned Carnivore-Paleo diet and a sustainable exercise program paves the path towards achieving and maintaining a healthy weight while simultaneously enhancing your overall well-being. This

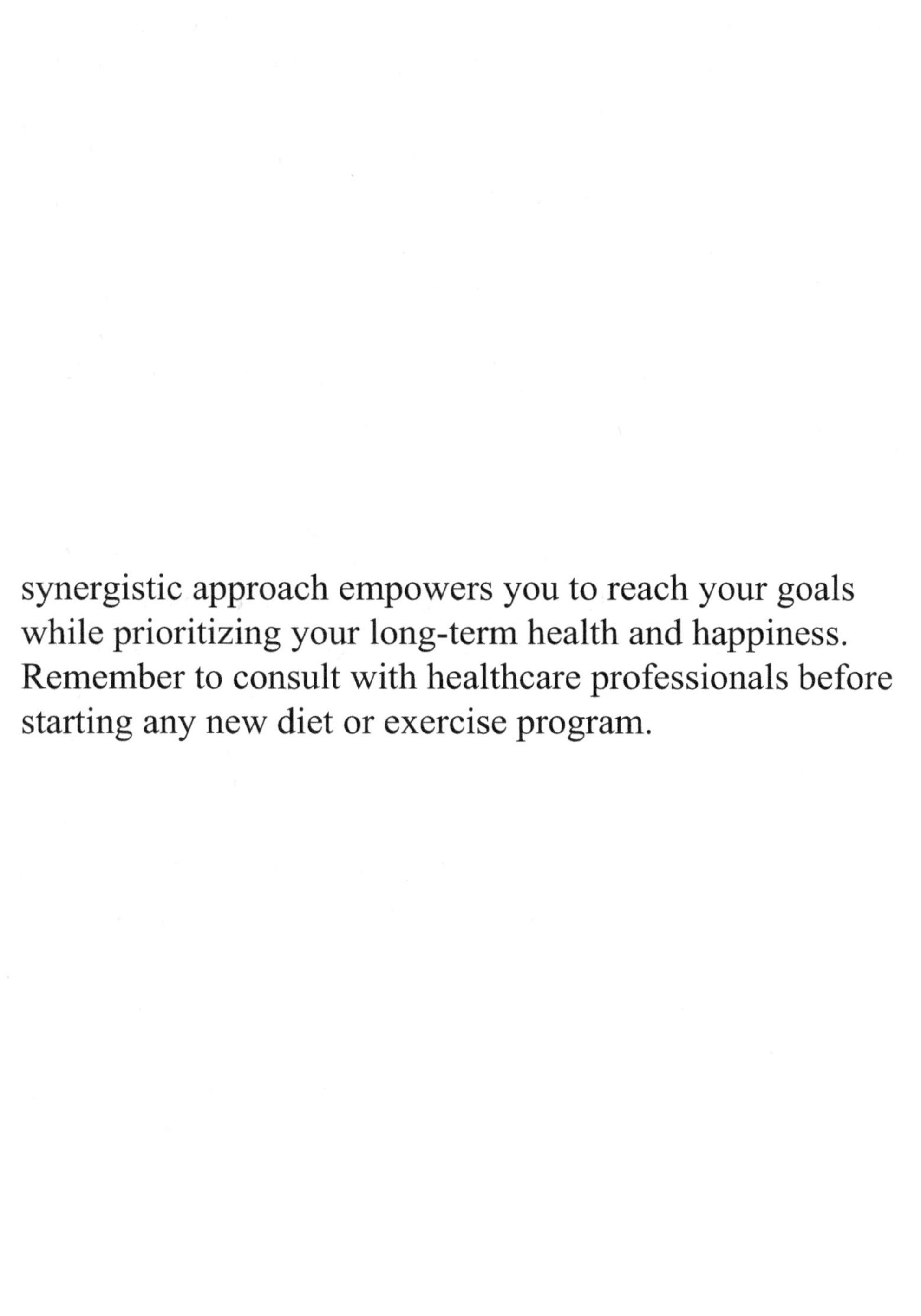

synergistic approach empowers you to reach your goals while prioritizing your long-term health and happiness. Remember to consult with healthcare professionals before starting any new diet or exercise program.

Walking Strength Training HIIT

Finding the right type of exercise is crucial for long-term success. It's not about punishing yourself; it's about finding activities you genuinely enjoy and can realistically incorporate into your lifestyle. The goal isn't to become a marathon runner overnight, but to gradually increase your activity levels and find sustainable routines that fit seamlessly into your daily life. This chapter explores three readily accessible and effective options: walking, strength training, and high-intensity interval training (HIIT). Let's delve into each one, highlighting its benefits and how to get started.

Walking is often overlooked as a form of exercise, but its simplicity and accessibility make it an excellent starting point for anyone, regardless of their fitness level. It requires no special equipment, can be done virtually anywhere, and can be easily integrated into your daily routine. A brisk walk for 30 minutes most days of the week can significantly improve your cardiovascular health, boost your mood, and contribute to weight loss. Start with shorter walks if needed, gradually increasing the duration and intensity as your fitness improves. Explore different routes to keep things interesting—walk in a park, along a scenic trail, or even around your neighborhood. Listen to your favorite podcast or audiobook to make the time more enjoyable. Consider investing in a pedometer or fitness tracker to monitor your steps and progress. Remember that consistency is key; even short, regular walks are more beneficial than sporadic, strenuous workouts.

Beyond the physical benefits, walking offers a valuable mental respite. It provides an opportunity to disconnect from the stresses of daily life and reconnect with yourself and your surroundings. The rhythmic movement can be meditative, allowing your mind to wander and clear itself of clutter. This mindful aspect of walking complements the focus on holistic well-being promoted by the Carnivore-Paleo approach. It's not just about burning calories; it's about nurturing your mental and emotional health. To further enhance the experience, consider incorporating mindful walking techniques, focusing on your breath and the sensation of your feet hitting the ground.

Strength training, often underestimated in its weight loss benefits, is a crucial component of a comprehensive fitness plan. It involves using resistance to build and maintain muscle mass. Muscle tissue is metabolically active, meaning it burns more calories even at rest. By increasing your muscle mass, you'll boost your metabolism and create a more efficient calorie-burning machine. Strength training also improves bone density, reducing the risk of osteoporosis, especially important as we age. It enhances posture, balance, and overall functional strength, making everyday tasks easier and reducing the risk of injuries. You don't need a gym membership to start strength training. Bodyweight exercises like squats, push-ups, lunges, and planks are effective and can be done at home with minimal equipment.

Beginners should start with a basic routine, focusing on proper form over the number of repetitions. Consult online resources, fitness apps, or a personal trainer for guidance on proper techniques. Start with two or three sessions per week, allowing for adequate rest between workouts. As you get stronger, you can gradually increase the intensity by adding more weight, repetitions, or sets. Consider investing in a set of resistance bands or dumbbells for added resistance. Remember to listen to your body and avoid pushing yourself too hard, especially when starting. Progressive overload is key—gradually increasing the challenge over time—to continually stimulate muscle growth and avoid plateaus.

High-Intensity Interval Training (HIIT) is a time-efficient workout method that alternates between short bursts of intense exercise and brief recovery periods. A typical HIIT session might involve 30 seconds of intense activity followed by 30 seconds of rest, repeated for 15-20 minutes. This type of training is highly effective for improving cardiovascular fitness, burning calories, and increasing metabolism. The intense bursts of activity stimulate your body's fat-burning processes, while the recovery periods allow for efficient oxygen replenishment. HIIT can be adapted to a wide range of activities, including running, cycling, jumping jacks, burpees, and other bodyweight exercises.

The beauty of HIIT lies in its flexibility. You can tailor the exercises to your fitness level and preferences. Beginners should start with shorter intervals and more frequent rest periods, gradually increasing the intensity and duration as their fitness improves. It's important to ensure proper warm-up and cool-down periods to prevent injuries. Remember that HIIT workouts are highly demanding, so listen to your body and take rest days when needed. Consistency is key, but overtraining can lead to injury and burnout. If you find HIIT too intense, consider modifying the exercises or reducing the duration of the high-intensity bursts. Ultimately, the goal is to find an exercise routine that you can maintain long-term without compromising your health and well-being.

Regardless of your chosen exercise type, remember to listen to your body. Don't push yourself too hard, especially when starting. Pain is a signal that something is wrong, so stop and rest if you experience any discomfort. Start slowly and gradually increase the intensity and duration of your workouts. Consistency is more important than intensity; short, regular workouts are more effective than sporadic, strenuous sessions. Remember to stay hydrated by drinking plenty of water before, during, and after your workouts. And most importantly, choose activities you enjoy. If you find exercise boring or unpleasant, you're less likely to stick with it. Find something that you genuinely look forward to, whether it's walking in nature, lifting weights, or participating in a group fitness class.

The Carnivore-Paleo approach emphasizes a holistic lifestyle, and exercise is an integral part of that. By incorporating regular physical activity, you'll not only enhance your weight loss efforts but also improve your overall health and well-being. This holistic perspective emphasizes the interconnectedness of physical activity, nutrition, and mental health. It's not just about achieving a specific weight; it's about nurturing your body and mind to reach your full potential.

Remember to consult with your healthcare provider or a qualified fitness professional before starting any new exercise program, especially if you have any underlying health conditions. They can help you create a personalized plan that meets your individual needs and goals, ensuring you're exercising safely and effectively. They can also address any concerns you might have about incorporating exercise into your routine. A professional can offer guidance on proper techniques, workout schedules, and modifications for specific needs.

Incorporating exercise into your lifestyle should be a gradual and enjoyable process. Don't strive for perfection; aim for progress. Celebrate your small victories, acknowledge your efforts, and appreciate the positive changes in your overall health and well-being. Remember that consistency is key, and finding activities you enjoy is crucial for long-term success. By embracing this holistic approach, you'll not only achieve your weight loss goals but also cultivate a healthier and more fulfilling lifestyle. The journey towards a healthier you is a marathon, not a sprint. Embrace the process, enjoy the journey, and celebrate your achievements along the way. The combination of a nutrient-dense Carnivore-Paleo diet and a consistent exercise program will empower you to achieve sustainable weight loss and a healthier, more energetic life. This approach prioritizes long-term well-being over quick fixes, fostering a sustainable lifestyle change that will benefit you for years to come. Remember, consistency and enjoyment are the keys to long-term success in any weight loss journey.

Creating a Sustainable Exercise Plan

Creating a truly sustainable exercise plan hinges on understanding your individual needs, preferences, and limitations. It's not a one-size-fits-all approach; what works wonders for one person might feel overwhelming or even counterproductive for another. The key is personalization, starting small, and gradually building up intensity and duration. This isn't about pushing yourself to the brink of exhaustion; it's about creating a routine that integrates seamlessly into your life, fostering a positive and long-lasting relationship with physical activity.

First, let's address the common hurdle of finding the time. Many people believe that a demanding exercise regimen requires hours each day, a misconception that often leads to discouragement before even beginning. The truth is, even short bursts of activity throughout the day can significantly contribute to overall fitness. Consider incorporating short walks during your lunch break, taking the stairs instead of the elevator, or engaging in quick bursts of bodyweight exercises during TV commercial breaks. These small, consistent efforts accumulate over time, leading to substantial improvements in fitness and well-being.

Next, consider your personal preferences. Do you find solace in the solitude of a solitary walk in nature, or do you thrive in the energetic atmosphere of a group fitness class? Do you prefer the structured routine of strength training or the cardiovascular benefits of running or swimming? Identifying your preferred activities is crucial; the more enjoyable an activity, the more likely you are to stick with it. Experiment with different options, exploring various types of exercise until you find those that genuinely resonate with you. Don't be afraid to try something new, even if you're initially hesitant. You might discover a hidden talent or a newfound passion that enriches your life.

The initial stages of any new exercise program should be focused on building a solid foundation. Start slowly and gradually increase the intensity and duration of your workouts. If you're new to exercise, begin with short walks for 15-20 minutes a few times a week. As your fitness level improves, gradually increase the duration and intensity of your walks, perhaps incorporating some gentle hills or a faster pace. Remember, consistency is more important than intensity, particularly in the initial phases. It's better to engage in regular, moderate activity than to sporadically push yourself too hard, risking injury and burnout.

Building a sustainable exercise plan also requires setting realistic goals. Avoid the trap of setting overly ambitious targets that can lead to discouragement and ultimately abandonment of the program. Instead, focus on setting small, achievable goals that gradually build upon each other. For instance, aim to walk for 30 minutes three times a week for the first month, then gradually increase the duration or frequency of your walks in subsequent months. Celebrate your achievements along the way, acknowledging the progress you've made, no matter how small. This positive reinforcement will help you stay motivated and committed to your fitness journey.

Tracking your progress is another essential component of a sustainable exercise plan. Keeping a journal or using a fitness app can help you monitor your workouts, track your progress, and stay accountable. This allows you to visualize your achievements, which is a powerful motivator. Seeing how far you've come can boost your confidence and encourage you to continue your efforts. Additionally, regularly reviewing your progress can help you identify areas for improvement and adjust your plan accordingly.

This ensures your program remains challenging yet achievable.

Integrating exercise into your routine necessitates strategic planning. Schedule your workouts just like you would any other important appointment. Treating exercise as a non-negotiable commitment helps ensure consistency. Find convenient times that work best for your schedule, whether it's early morning, lunchtime, or evening. If you struggle to find dedicated time, incorporate short bursts of activity into your daily life, such as taking the stairs instead of the elevator or walking during your lunch break. These small changes accumulate to provide significant benefits.

Finding an exercise buddy can also significantly boost motivation and adherence. Having someone to exercise with provides accountability, encouragement, and shared motivation. Moreover, exercising with a friend or family member can make the process more enjoyable, helping you stay committed to your fitness goals. If you find it challenging to motivate yourself, consider joining a group fitness class or finding a workout partner who shares your goals and fitness level.

Nutrition plays a crucial role in supporting your exercise program. Ensure you're consuming a sufficient amount of nutrients to fuel your workouts and aid recovery. The Carnivore-Paleo approach provides a foundation for this; the nutrient-dense nature of the foods supports muscle growth and repair, energy production, and overall well-being. Adequate hydration is also essential for optimal performance and recovery. Make sure you're drinking plenty of water throughout the day, especially before, during, and after your workouts.

It's essential to listen to your body and rest when needed. Overtraining can lead to injury, burnout, and derail your progress. Incorporate rest days into your exercise plan to allow your body to recover and rebuild. Don't hesitate to modify or even skip a workout if you're feeling unwell or excessively fatigued. Prioritizing rest and recovery is just as important as the exercise itself. This holistic approach to fitness ensures long-term sustainability and minimizes the risk of injury.

Variety is another key to a sustainable exercise routine. Avoid monotony by incorporating different types of exercise into your program. This keeps your workouts fresh and engaging, preventing boredom and reducing the likelihood of quitting. Mix up your routine by trying different activities, exploring new locations, or varying the intensity of your workouts. This ensures that your body continues to adapt and improve, maximizing the overall benefits of your exercise program. Remember, exercise shouldn't feel like a chore; it should be an enjoyable part of your life.

Finally, remember that setbacks are a normal part of any fitness journey. Don't let occasional lapses in your routine derail your progress. If you miss a workout or have a less-than-ideal day, simply pick yourself up, dust yourself off, and get back on track. The key is consistency and perseverance, not perfection. Focus on the long-term goals and celebrate your successes along the way. Creating a sustainable exercise plan is a personal journey; find what works best for you, and adapt your plan as needed. With patience, perseverance, and a focus on long-term consistency, you'll not only achieve your fitness goals but also cultivate a healthier, more energetic, and fulfilling life.

Listening to Your Body

The previous chapter emphasized the importance of finding an exercise routine that fits seamlessly into your life, focusing on consistency over intensity. However, even the most carefully crafted plan can backfire if you neglect the crucial element of rest and recovery. Overtraining is a significant risk, not just for hindering weight loss progress but also for jeopardizing your overall health and well-being. It's a common pitfall, especially when initial enthusiasm leads to pushing your body beyond its capacity. This section will delve into recognizing the signs of overtraining, understanding the importance of rest days, and developing strategies to ensure your exercise routine supports, rather than sabotages, your health goals.

The human body isn't a machine; it requires time to repair and rebuild itself after physical stress. Exercise, while beneficial, places demands on your muscles, bones, tendons, and ligaments. These tissues undergo microscopic damage during workouts, and it's during the rest periods that they repair themselves, becoming stronger and more resilient. When you consistently push your body without adequate recovery, you enter the realm of overtraining. This isn't simply about feeling tired; it's a state of chronic fatigue that impacts your physical and mental well-being in several ways.

One of the most noticeable signs of overtraining is persistent fatigue, extending far beyond the normal tiredness experienced after a strenuous workout. This fatigue isn't alleviated by sleep or rest; it lingers, impacting your daily activities and mood. You might find yourself struggling to perform even simple tasks, feeling perpetually sluggish and lacking energy. This persistent exhaustion is a significant red flag, indicating that your body needs a break.

Beyond fatigue, overtraining often manifests as decreased performance. If you find that your workouts are becoming increasingly difficult, even though you're maintaining the same routine, it could be a sign that your body is struggling to keep up. Your strength, endurance, and overall athletic performance may decline despite your consistent efforts. This is a clear indication that your body isn't recovering adequately, and you need to adjust your training regimen.

Another crucial indicator is increased susceptibility to illness. When your body is constantly stressed from overtraining, your immune system weakens, making you more vulnerable to infections. Frequent colds, flu, or other illnesses are a warning sign that your body is struggling to cope with the demands placed upon it. This weakened immune response underscores the importance of rest in maintaining a strong and resilient immune system.

Beyond the physical symptoms, overtraining can significantly impact your mental health. You may experience increased irritability, mood swings, difficulty concentrating, and even symptoms of depression or anxiety. This mental fatigue is linked to the physical exhaustion and the overall stress on your system. Ignoring these mental signs is a mistake, as mental well-being is inextricably linked to physical health.

Sleep disturbances are another common symptom. Even when you sleep for what seems like adequate time, you might experience restless nights, difficulty falling asleep, or waking up feeling unrefreshed. This sleep disruption is a consequence of the chronic stress placed on your body and mind. Addressing sleep issues is crucial in managing overtraining and ensuring your body has the opportunity to repair itself.

Muscle soreness is expected after a workout, but persistent, excessive muscle soreness that doesn't subside with rest is a red flag. This is particularly true if the soreness is accompanied by other symptoms like fatigue, decreased performance, and increased susceptibility to illness. Prolonged muscle soreness suggests your muscles are not recovering properly and need a longer period of rest.

Changes in appetite are also worth noting. Significant changes—either a dramatic increase or decrease in appetite—can signal overtraining. This can be caused by hormonal imbalances or the body's attempt to conserve energy due to excessive stress. Paying attention to your appetite can offer valuable insights into your body's overall state.

What constitutes "overtraining" is subjective and varies depending on individual factors such as fitness level, training intensity, and overall health. A beginner's definition of overtraining will differ significantly from that of a seasoned athlete. Therefore, it's crucial to listen to your body and be aware of your own individual responses. There is no one-size-fits-all answer, and a personalized approach is essential.

Listening to your body involves paying close attention to the signals it sends. This goes beyond simply acknowledging physical symptoms; it's about developing an intuitive understanding of your body's needs. This means being attuned to subtle changes in your energy levels, mood, appetite, and sleep patterns. Take the time to reflect on how you feel after each workout, noting both physical and emotional responses. Regular self-assessment is crucial in preventing overtraining.

Rest days are not lazy days; they are essential components of a successful fitness plan. Scheduled rest periods allow your body to repair and rebuild, preventing injury and promoting progress. While the frequency of rest days varies depending on individual needs and training intensity, incorporating at least one or two rest days per week is generally recommended. On these days, avoid strenuous activities, opting instead for light, restorative activities like gentle walking or stretching.

Consider active recovery strategies on your rest days. Instead of complete inactivity, engage in low-intensity activities like yoga, Pilates, or a leisurely walk. These activities promote blood flow, improve flexibility, and reduce muscle soreness without placing additional strain on your body. Active recovery can aid in the recovery process while still keeping your body moving.

Prioritize sleep. Aim for 7-9 hours of quality sleep each night. Sleep is the body's primary time for repair and restoration. Establish a regular sleep schedule, create a relaxing bedtime routine, and optimize your sleep environment to ensure you get the rest you need. Consistent, quality sleep is critical for physical and mental recovery.

Proper nutrition plays a vital role in preventing overtraining. Ensure you're consuming a balanced diet rich in protein, healthy fats, and essential nutrients. The Carnivore-Paleo approach, as detailed in previous chapters, provides a solid foundation for nutrient-dense meals, supporting muscle repair and overall recovery. Focus on nutrient timing, consuming sufficient protein after your workouts to promote muscle growth and repair. Adequate hydration is equally important for optimal bodily function and recovery.

Hydration is often overlooked but is crucial for recovery. Water helps regulate body temperature, transport nutrients, and remove waste products from your muscles. Dehydration can significantly impair performance and recovery. Aim to drink plenty of water throughout the day, especially before, during, and after your workouts.

Stress management is also an integral part of preventing overtraining. Chronic stress can exacerbate fatigue and impair recovery. Incorporate stress-reducing techniques into your routine, such as meditation, deep breathing exercises, or spending time in nature. These practices promote relaxation and help your body cope with the demands of exercise. Mindfulness practices can be particularly helpful in tuning into your body's signals and responding appropriately.

Listen to your body. Don't push through pain or extreme fatigue. Learning to distinguish between normal muscle soreness and pain that signals an injury is vital. If you experience sharp or persistent pain, stop the activity and seek professional medical advice. Ignoring pain can lead to more severe injuries, setting you back significantly.

Seek professional guidance. Consult with a qualified healthcare professional or certified personal trainer who can create a personalized exercise plan tailored to your individual needs and goals. Regular check-ins with a trainer can help you monitor your progress and make necessary adjustments to prevent overtraining. A professional's guidance can help you avoid common pitfalls and optimize your fitness journey.

Flexibility is key. Don't be afraid to modify your exercise plan based on your body's response. If you're feeling overly fatigued or experiencing symptoms of overtraining, reduce the intensity or duration of your workouts, or take additional rest days. A flexible approach allows you to adapt to your changing needs and prevent burnout. It's a sign of intelligence, not weakness, to modify your approach when necessary.

In conclusion, incorporating exercise into your routine is crucial for weight loss and overall health. However, a balanced approach that prioritizes rest and recovery is just as important. Overtraining is a real risk, but by carefully listening to your body, respecting rest days, prioritizing sleep and nutrition, and managing stress, you can create a sustainable exercise routine that supports your goals without jeopardizing your well-being. Remember that progress is not always linear; setbacks are part of the journey, and listening to your body is the key to achieving long-term success. Don't strive for perfection; strive for consistency and mindful adaptation.

Integrating Exercise with Your Diet

Building a successful weight loss journey using the Carnivore-Paleo approach requires a holistic strategy that integrates mindful eating with regular physical activity. The synergistic effect of these two components is far greater than the sum of their parts. While the dietary aspect focuses on providing your body with nutrient-dense foods to fuel your metabolism and support optimal function, exercise enhances calorie expenditure, builds muscle mass, and improves overall body composition. The key is to find a balance that works for you, avoiding the pitfalls of overtraining while maximizing the benefits of both diet and exercise.

Let's start by addressing a common misconception: exercise doesn't simply burn calories; it's a powerful catalyst for metabolic changes. When you engage in regular physical activity, particularly resistance training, your body increases its resting metabolic rate (RMR). This means you burn more calories even when you're at rest. This effect is amplified when combined with a Carnivore-Paleo diet, which naturally boosts metabolism due to its high protein and healthy fat content. Protein requires more energy to digest than carbohydrates, further enhancing the caloric expenditure.

The type of exercise you choose is crucial. While high-intensity interval training (HIIT) is highly effective for calorie burning, it shouldn't be the only form of exercise in your routine. HIIT can be extremely demanding, and incorporating it without sufficient rest and recovery can lead to burnout and injury. A well-rounded exercise plan should include a variety of activities to target different muscle groups and improve overall fitness.

Consider incorporating strength training, which is especially beneficial when following a high-protein diet. Building muscle mass not only improves your physique but also significantly increases your RMR. Even small increases in muscle mass can lead to substantial long-term calorie burning. Beginners can start with bodyweight exercises like squats, push-ups, and lunges. As you progress, you can incorporate weights or resistance bands to progressively overload your muscles.

Cardiovascular exercise, such as brisk walking, jogging, swimming, or cycling, is equally important for cardiovascular health and overall well-being. These activities help improve heart function, reduce stress, and contribute to overall calorie expenditure. The key is to find an activity you enjoy, making it sustainable in the long run. Don't force yourself into activities you dislike; this will only lead to frustration and a lack of consistency.

Flexibility and balance exercises, often neglected, are essential components of a comprehensive fitness plan. Yoga, Pilates, and Tai Chi improve flexibility, balance, and coordination, reducing the risk of injuries and improving overall body awareness. These activities are particularly beneficial as we age, helping to maintain mobility and prevent falls.

The timing of your exercise in relation to your meals is also a factor to consider. Some people find that exercising in a fasted state (before eating) enhances fat burning. However, others perform better with a light snack or meal beforehand to provide sufficient energy for their workout. Experiment to see what works best for your body and energy levels. Listen to your body's signals; if you feel weak or lightheaded during exercise, stop and have a small, nutrient-dense snack.

Hydration is paramount during exercise. Dehydration can lead to fatigue, muscle cramps, and reduced performance. Ensure you drink plenty of water throughout the day, especially before, during, and after your workout.

Electrolytes are also important, especially during prolonged or intense exercise. Natural sources of electrolytes like bone broth can be beneficial.

Monitoring your progress is essential to stay motivated and adjust your exercise routine as needed. Track your workouts, noting the types of exercise you've done, the duration, and the intensity. You can also use a fitness tracker or app to monitor your heart rate, steps, and calories burned. However, remember that these tools are merely aids; the most important measure is how you feel. Focus on improvements in your strength, endurance, and overall well-being rather than solely focusing on numbers.

Integrating exercise into your Carnivore-Paleo lifestyle shouldn't feel like a chore. Find activities that you genuinely enjoy and that fit seamlessly into your schedule. If you struggle to find time for dedicated workouts, consider incorporating movement into your daily routine. Take the stairs instead of the elevator, walk or cycle instead of driving short distances, and stand up regularly if you have a sedentary job. These small changes can accumulate over time and contribute significantly to your overall calorie expenditure and fitness level.

Remember, consistency is key. It's better to engage in moderate exercise most days of the week than to push yourself too hard a few days and then burn out. Listen to your body; rest when you need to, and don't be afraid to adjust your exercise plan based on your progress and energy levels. Don't compare yourself to others; everyone's journey is unique.

Furthermore, consider the impact of stress on your weight loss efforts. Chronic stress can lead to increased cortisol levels, which can promote fat storage, particularly around the abdomen. Incorporate stress-reducing activities into your routine, such as meditation, yoga, spending time in nature, or engaging in hobbies you enjoy. Adequate sleep is also crucial; aim for 7-9 hours of quality sleep per night to allow your body to recover and repair itself.

The combination of a well-planned Carnivore-Paleo diet and a sustainable exercise routine is a powerful strategy for achieving long-term weight loss and improved health. It's a journey, not a race. Celebrate your successes, learn from your setbacks, and remember that consistency, not perfection, is the key to sustainable results. By prioritizing your overall well-being and finding activities that you enjoy, you can build a healthy lifestyle that supports your weight loss goals and enhances your quality of life. This holistic approach—combining mindful eating with enjoyable exercise and stress management—sets you up for sustained success, empowering you to achieve your health and fitness aspirations.

Remember to consult with your doctor or a qualified healthcare professional before starting any new diet or exercise program, especially if you have any underlying health conditions. They can help you personalize a plan that's safe and effective for your individual needs and circumstances. They can also monitor your progress and address any concerns you may have. This collaborative approach will ensure your journey to a healthier lifestyle is both safe and successful. Don't hesitate to seek professional guidance; it's an investment in your long-term health and well-being. The support of a healthcare professional can make all the difference in achieving your goals and maintaining a healthy lifestyle for years to come. This proactive approach underscores the importance of personalized care in achieving sustainable weight loss and overall wellness.

The Role of Sleep in Weight Management

Sleep, often overlooked in the pursuit of weight loss, plays a surprisingly crucial role in your journey towards a healthier, slimmer you. While diet and exercise are cornerstones of weight management, neglecting sleep undermines your efforts and can even sabotage your progress. This is because sleep profoundly influences several physiological processes directly impacting weight regulation.

First, let's consider the hormones governing appetite and satiety. Leptin and ghrelin are two key players in this hormonal dance. Leptin, produced by fat cells, signals to your brain that you're full. Ghrelin, on the other hand, is your hunger hormone, stimulating appetite. Insufficient sleep disrupts this delicate balance, suppressing leptin production and simultaneously increasing ghrelin levels. The result? You feel less satisfied after meals and experience heightened hunger, making it significantly harder to maintain a calorie deficit. Imagine the frustration of meticulously tracking your macros, exercising diligently, yet constantly battling overwhelming cravings due to sleep deprivation. This hormonal imbalance can easily derail even the most well-intentioned weight loss plans.

Furthermore, sleep deprivation impacts your metabolism. Studies consistently demonstrate a link between insufficient sleep and a slowed metabolic rate. Your body burns fewer calories at rest when sleep-deprived, essentially making it harder to shed those extra pounds. This metabolic slowdown isn't simply a minor inconvenience; it's a significant obstacle. The cumulative effect of a consistently slower metabolism over weeks and months can result in substantial weight gain, even with a relatively controlled diet. This metabolic disruption also influences insulin sensitivity – your body's ability to effectively utilize glucose. Poor sleep can lead to insulin resistance, further contributing to weight gain and increasing the risk of developing type 2 diabetes.

Beyond the metabolic and hormonal impacts, sleep deprivation affects your willpower and decision-making. When sleep-deprived, your prefrontal cortex – the brain region responsible for executive functions like self-control and impulse control – functions less effectively. This impaired cognitive function makes it more challenging to resist unhealthy food choices, especially those high in sugar and fat, which offer a temporary mood boost. The late-night cravings, impulsive snacking, and the overall lack of self-discipline often associated with sleep deprivation can significantly hinder your weight loss progress. It's a vicious cycle: poor sleep leads to poor choices, leading to further weight gain, leading to even poorer sleep.

Consider the stress response. When sleep-deprived, your body is in a constant state of mild stress. This chronic low-grade stress elevates cortisol levels, the infamous "stress hormone". High cortisol levels not only increase appetite but also promote fat storage, particularly around the abdomen. This abdominal fat is often associated with increased health risks, making sleep a crucial factor not just for weight management, but for overall well-being. The combination of increased appetite, impaired decision-making, and fat storage driven by chronic stress induced by lack of sleep makes it almost impossible to achieve or maintain a healthy weight.

The impact of sleep extends beyond these immediate physiological consequences. Adequate sleep improves your mood, energy levels, and overall sense of well-being. These factors are essential for maintaining motivation and adherence to your weight loss plan. Feeling constantly tired and irritable makes it far more likely to abandon your healthy eating habits and exercise routine. A well-rested individual is better equipped to handle the challenges and temptations that inevitably arise during a weight loss journey.

Now, let's look at practical steps to improve your sleep quality. The first, and perhaps most significant, step is establishing a regular sleep schedule. Go to bed and wake up around the same time each day, even on weekends, to regulate your body's natural sleep-wake cycle. This consistency is key to optimizing your circadian rhythm, a crucial aspect of healthy sleep. Think of it as training your body to expect sleep at a specific time. Avoid inconsistent sleep patterns; they're detrimental to sleep quality and hormonal balance.

Creating a relaxing bedtime routine is another powerful tool. This routine could involve a warm bath, reading a book (avoid screens!), listening to calming music, or practicing gentle stretching or yoga. These activities signal to your body that it's time to wind down and prepare for sleep. Avoid stimulating activities like intense workouts or screen time (phones, tablets, computers, and televisions) close to bedtime. The blue light emitted from these devices interferes with melatonin production, a hormone essential for regulating sleep. Many find that even an hour before bed, screen time should be avoided.

Optimize your sleep environment. Ensure your bedroom is dark, quiet, and cool. Invest in comfortable bedding, blackout curtains if needed, and earplugs to minimize light and noise distractions. A consistently cool room is optimal for sleep; your body naturally lowers its temperature in preparation for sleep. A comfortable mattress and pillows are investments in better sleep, and hence, better health. These environmental factors significantly impact sleep quality and can make a world of difference.

Consider your diet and hydration. While we've emphasized the role of sleep in weight management, the reverse is also true. A late-night heavy meal can disrupt your sleep. Similarly, consuming excessive caffeine or alcohol before bed can interfere with sleep quality. Staying well-hydrated is vital for overall health, but excessive water intake close to bedtime may lead to frequent nighttime bathroom trips, disrupting sleep. Mindful hydration during the day but limiting fluid intake close to bedtime can greatly improve your quality of sleep.

Addressing stress is crucial for better sleep. Stress is a significant sleep disruptor. If stress is impacting your sleep, explore stress management techniques like meditation, deep breathing exercises, yoga, spending time in nature, or engaging in hobbies you enjoy. These practices promote relaxation and help you manage the physical and mental symptoms of stress. Finding ways to alleviate chronic stress is paramount for achieving and maintaining restful sleep. Remember, chronic stress is a significant contributor to poor sleep and weight gain.

If you've tried these strategies and still struggle with sleep, consult a healthcare professional. Underlying sleep disorders such as sleep apnea or insomnia can significantly impact weight management. A doctor can help identify and address any underlying medical conditions interfering with your sleep. Addressing any such problems is essential for overall health and weight management. Don't underestimate the importance of seeking professional help if necessary.

In summary, prioritizing sleep is not a luxury, but a necessity in your weight loss journey. It's a cornerstone of metabolic health, hormonal balance, and effective stress management. By incorporating the practical strategies outlined above, you can significantly improve your sleep quality, leading to better overall health and easier weight management. Remember, a well-rested body is a body better equipped to achieve its weight loss goals. Consistent sleep is an essential, non-negotiable component of a successful, sustainable weight loss plan. Don't underestimate its power.

Strategies for Improving Sleep Quality

Building upon the crucial role of sleep in weight management, let's delve into practical strategies to optimize your sleep quality. While prioritizing sleep might seem like a secondary concern compared to diet and exercise, its impact on your weight loss journey is profound and often underestimated. Poor sleep disrupts hormonal balance, increases cravings, and reduces energy levels, making it harder to stick to your healthy eating plan and exercise routine.

One of the most effective ways to improve sleep quality is to establish a regular sleep schedule. This means going to bed and waking up around the same time every day, even on weekends. Consistency is key; it helps regulate your body's natural sleep-wake cycle, known as your circadian rhythm. This rhythm dictates when you feel sleepy and when you feel alert, and disrupting it can lead to sleep disturbances and daytime fatigue. Think of it as training your body to anticipate sleep at a specific time, making the transition into slumber smoother and more efficient. Aim for 7-9 hours of sleep per night, a range widely recommended for optimal health and well-being.

Creating a relaxing bedtime routine is equally crucial. This routine should be a consistent sequence of calming activities that signal to your body that it's time to wind down. Avoid screen time at least an hour before bed, as the blue light emitted from electronic devices interferes with melatonin production, a hormone essential for regulating sleep. Instead, opt for relaxing activities like reading a physical book, taking a warm bath, listening to soothing music, or practicing gentle stretching or yoga. These activities help reduce stress and anxiety, paving the way for better sleep. Experiment with different activities to find what works best for you, aiming to create a personalized routine that you genuinely enjoy and look forward to each night.

Optimizing your sleep environment is another critical step towards better sleep. Your bedroom should be dark, quiet, and cool. Invest in blackout curtains or an eye mask to block out light, and consider using earplugs to minimize noise distractions. A comfortable mattress and pillows are also vital; ensure your bedding is supportive and conducive to restful sleep. Maintaining a consistently cool room temperature, around 65 degrees Fahrenheit (18 degrees Celsius), is often ideal for sleep. A cool environment helps regulate your body temperature, which naturally drops slightly as you prepare for sleep. The room should also be well-ventilated to ensure fresh air circulation. Clutter can also affect your sleep, so keeping your bedroom tidy and organized can contribute to a more peaceful sleep environment.

Beyond these environmental factors, dietary choices can significantly impact sleep quality. While the Carnivore-Paleo approach generally promotes healthy sleep due to its focus on nutrient-dense, whole foods, certain dietary considerations are still relevant. Avoid heavy meals or large amounts of caffeine or alcohol close to bedtime. Heavy meals can interfere with digestion and lead to discomfort that disrupts sleep. Caffeine is a stimulant that can keep you awake, and even a small amount consumed later in the day can affect sleep quality. Alcohol, though initially sedative, can disrupt sleep cycles later in the night, leading to poor-quality rest. Consider having a lighter dinner earlier in the evening, focusing on easily digestible proteins and vegetables. A small bedtime snack, such as a small handful of nuts or a piece of cheese, might be helpful for some individuals, but it's crucial to experiment and find what works best for you without causing digestive discomfort. Sufficient hydration throughout the day is also essential, but avoid excessive fluid intake close to bedtime to minimize nighttime bathroom trips.

Stress and anxiety are major sleep disruptors. Managing stress effectively is, therefore, crucial for improving sleep quality. Various techniques can help you reduce stress levels. Regular exercise is a powerful stress reliever, but it's crucial to avoid intense workouts right before bed. Instead, engage in moderate exercise earlier in the day. Mindfulness and meditation techniques, even for short periods, can significantly reduce stress and promote relaxation. Deep breathing exercises are particularly helpful in calming the nervous system before bedtime. Progressive muscle relaxation, a technique involving systematically tensing and releasing different muscle groups, can also relieve tension and promote relaxation. Consider incorporating these stress-management techniques into your daily routine, ideally as part of your relaxing bedtime routine.

Furthermore, addressing underlying medical conditions can play a crucial role in improving sleep. If you consistently experience sleep problems despite following good sleep hygiene practices, consult your physician or a sleep specialist. Various medical conditions, such as sleep apnea, restless legs syndrome, and thyroid disorders, can contribute to sleep disturbances. A proper diagnosis and appropriate treatment can significantly improve your sleep quality. Addressing any underlying medical issues is crucial for obtaining a restful night's sleep.

Beyond these practical tips, exploring the power of sunlight exposure during the day can significantly enhance your sleep patterns. Sunlight exposure helps regulate your circadian rhythm by suppressing melatonin production in the morning and promoting its production in the evening. Aim for at least 15-30 minutes of sunlight exposure each day, especially in the morning. This natural light exposure helps synchronize your body's internal clock, leading to improved sleep-wake cycles. Combined with a consistent sleep schedule, this becomes a powerful tool to optimize your sleep patterns.

Finally, remember that consistency is paramount. Improving sleep quality isn't a one-time fix; it's a process that requires consistent effort and dedication. Don't get discouraged if you don't see results immediately. Continue implementing these strategies, and over time, you'll likely experience significant improvements in your sleep quality. Track your sleep patterns using a sleep tracker or simply by noting how you feel each day. This allows you to observe the effects of your changes, adjust your approach as needed, and celebrate your progress. Remember, improved sleep quality translates into enhanced energy levels, improved mood, better cognitive function, and a stronger ability to stick to your weight loss goals. Prioritizing sleep is not a luxury; it's an essential investment in your overall health and well-being, directly contributing to your success on your weight loss journey. The impact of good sleep extends far beyond just feeling rested; it's fundamental to hormonal balance, appetite regulation, and efficient stress management—all crucial elements in achieving and maintaining a healthy weight. Don't underestimate the transformative power of a good night's sleep.

Understanding the Impact of Stress on Weight

The connection between stress and weight is undeniable, a complex interplay that often sabotages even the most diligently planned weight loss efforts. While we've explored the crucial role of sleep in optimizing your body's natural rhythms, understanding the impact of stress is equally vital. Stress, in its many forms – financial worries, relationship difficulties, work pressures, or even seemingly minor daily annoyances – triggers a cascade of hormonal responses that directly affect your metabolism, appetite, and overall well-being, often leading to weight gain.

One of the primary culprits is the hormone cortisol. When you're stressed, your body releases cortisol, often referred to as the "stress hormone." In short bursts, cortisol is beneficial; it helps you cope with immediate threats. However, chronic, elevated cortisol levels – a hallmark of ongoing stress – disrupt the delicate balance of your endocrine system. This disruption manifests in several ways detrimental to weight management.

Firstly, elevated cortisol promotes fat storage, particularly around the abdomen. This visceral fat, nestled deep within your abdominal cavity, is metabolically active, releasing inflammatory substances that negatively impact your health. It's not just about aesthetics; visceral fat increases the risk of heart disease, type 2 diabetes, and other chronic illnesses. The body prioritizes energy storage in these areas when cortisol levels remain high for extended periods, diverting resources away from other essential functions.

Secondly, cortisol impacts blood sugar regulation. Under stress, your body releases glucose into the bloodstream to provide quick energy for the "fight-or-flight" response. If you're not actively engaging in physical activity to utilize this extra glucose, it gets stored as fat. This explains why stress can lead to increased cravings for sugary and processed foods – your body craves quick energy to counteract the effects of stress, leading to a vicious cycle of stress-induced eating and subsequent weight gain. These cravings often target comfort foods rich in carbohydrates and fats, which provide a temporary sense of relief but ultimately contribute to weight gain.

Furthermore, stress impacts your gut microbiome. Emerging research increasingly highlights the crucial role of gut health in overall well-being, including weight management. Chronic stress disrupts the delicate balance of bacteria in your gut, potentially leading to inflammation and digestive issues that further complicate weight loss efforts. A healthy gut microbiome supports efficient digestion and nutrient absorption, and stress significantly undermines this critical function. This imbalance can lead to bloating, discomfort, and impaired nutrient absorption, potentially hindering your progress.

Beyond the physiological effects, stress also impacts your behavioral habits. When stressed, many individuals find solace in comfort eating, often turning to high-calorie, processed foods that provide temporary emotional relief. This stress-eating behavior can easily derail even the most meticulously planned dietary regimen. It's important to recognize this pattern and actively develop healthier coping mechanisms. Instead of reaching for unhealthy foods, consider engaging in activities that reduce stress, such as meditation, yoga, or spending time in nature.

Sleep deprivation, as discussed in the previous chapter, exacerbates the negative impact of stress. Lack of sleep further elevates cortisol levels, compounding the effects on your metabolism and appetite. When sleep-deprived and stressed, you are more susceptible to emotional eating and less likely to adhere to your healthy eating and exercise plans. This highlights the synergistic relationship between sleep and stress management in successful weight loss. Addressing both simultaneously is crucial for optimal results.

Effectively managing stress is, therefore, paramount for successful weight management. This doesn't involve eliminating stress entirely – that's simply unrealistic – but rather developing healthy coping mechanisms and strategies to mitigate its negative effects. Here's a range of techniques proven effective in reducing stress levels and supporting weight loss goals:

Mindfulness and Meditation:
Practicing mindfulness
involves focusing on the present moment, without judgment. Meditation, a core component of mindfulness, helps calm the mind, reduce anxiety, and lower cortisol levels. Even short, regular meditation sessions can have a profound impact on your stress levels and overall well-being. Many guided meditation apps are available to help you get started, offering a variety of techniques suited to different needs and experience levels.

Yoga and Deep Breathing Exercises:
Yoga combines physical postures, breathing techniques, and meditation to promote relaxation and stress reduction. Deep breathing exercises, a key element of yoga, can quickly calm your nervous system and reduce feelings of anxiety. Even a few minutes of deep, conscious breathing can make a noticeable difference. These techniques help regulate your autonomic nervous system, reducing the physiological impact of stress on your body.

Spending Time in Nature:
Studies have shown that
spending time outdoors, whether walking in a park or hiking
in the mountains, can significantly reduce stress levels.
Exposure to natural light and fresh air has a restorative effect
on both your mind and body. Connecting with nature
provides a natural escape from daily stressors and promotes
a sense of peace and calm.

Regular Exercise:
Physical activity is a highly effective stress reliever. Exercise
releases endorphins, natural mood boosters that alleviate
stress and improve overall well-being.
Choose activities you enjoy, whether it's brisk walking,
swimming, cycling, or strength training. The key is
consistency, finding activities that fit into your lifestyle and
that you can maintain over the long term.

Social Connection:
Strong social support networks are vital in managing stress.
Connecting with loved ones, engaging in social activities,
and fostering positive relationships can provide emotional
support and buffer against the negative effects of stress.
Feeling connected and supported reduces feelings of
isolation and helps you cope with challenging situations.

Time Management Techniques:
Effective time
management can reduce stress by creating a sense of control
and reducing feelings of being overwhelmed. Prioritize
tasks, break down large projects into smaller, manageable
steps, and learn to say no to commitments that add
unnecessary stress. This sense of control can significantly
impact your overall stress levels.

Cognitive Behavioral Therapy (CBT):
CBT is a form of psychotherapy that helps you identify
and change negative thought patterns and behaviors
contributing to stress and

anxiety. A trained therapist can guide you through techniques to challenge negative thoughts and develop more adaptive coping strategies. CBT can be particularly effective in addressing chronic stress and its impact on weight management.

Journaling:
Writing down your thoughts and feelings can be a powerful way to process stress and gain perspective.
Journaling helps you identify triggers, track your progress, and develop healthier coping mechanisms. It offers a safe space to express emotions without judgment, facilitating emotional regulation and stress reduction.

Professional Help:
If stress is significantly impacting your life and you're struggling to manage it on your own, don't hesitate to seek professional help. Therapists and counselors can provide guidance and support in developing effective coping strategies. They can help you address underlying issues contributing to your stress and develop personalized plans to manage stress effectively.

Remember, managing stress is not a one-size-fits-all approach. Experiment with different techniques to find what works best for you. The key is consistency and incorporating these strategies into your daily routine as an integral part of your overall well-being and successful weight management journey. By actively addressing stress, you are not only improving your mental and emotional health but also setting yourself up for long-term success in achieving and maintaining a healthy weight. Prioritizing stress management is an investment in your overall well-being, significantly contributing to a healthier, happier, and more fulfilling life. The journey to a healthy weight is not solely about diet and exercise; it's about cultivating a holistic approach that addresses the interconnectedness of mind, body, and spirit. By incorporating these stress-reducing strategies, you are not just managing weight, you are building a sustainable foundation for a healthier and more balanced life.

Effective Stress Management Techniques

Effective stress management is paramount for successful weight loss, particularly when following a Carnivore or Paleo approach. These diets, while beneficial for many, can sometimes be perceived as restrictive, potentially leading to stress if not approached with a mindful and balanced perspective. The stress response, characterized by the release of cortisol and other hormones, can disrupt metabolic processes, increase appetite, and even lead to cravings for less-than-ideal foods. Therefore, proactively managing stress is not just a supplementary element but a fundamental pillar of a successful weight-loss journey using these dietary approaches.

One highly effective technique is
meditation
. The practice of focusing on the present moment, often through
mindfulness exercises, can significantly reduce stress levels. Even short, 10-15 minute meditation sessions daily can have profound effects. There are numerous guided meditation apps available, making it easily accessible even for beginners. The goal isn't to clear your mind completely, but rather to acknowledge thoughts and feelings without judgment, letting them pass like clouds in the sky. This cultivates a sense of calm and mental clarity, reducing the reactivity that often accompanies stress. The regular practice of meditation helps to retrain your brain to respond to stressors in a more balanced and less reactive way. Over time, you'll find that you handle stressful situations with greater composure and resilience.

Complementary to meditation is the practice of
yoga
. This ancient discipline combines physical postures, breathing techniques (pranayama), and meditation to promote physical

and mental well-being. Yoga's gentle movements help release tension in the muscles, improve flexibility, and increase body awareness. The deep breathing exercises are particularly effective in calming the nervous system and lowering cortisol levels. While power yoga offers a vigorous workout, restorative yoga, with its emphasis on relaxation and prolonged holds, can be particularly beneficial for stress reduction. Even a short yoga session before bed can significantly improve sleep quality, further mitigating the effects of stress. Many free online yoga classes cater to different skill levels and preferences, making it an accessible option for everyone. The combination of physical movement and mindful breathing helps create a sense of groundedness and balance, countering the anxiety and tension often associated with stressful situations.

Deep breathing exercises
are simple yet powerful tools for stress management. These techniques can be practiced
anytime, anywhere, requiring no special equipment or settings. The most commonly used method is diaphragmatic breathing, also known as belly breathing. This technique involves inhaling deeply into your abdomen, allowing your belly to expand, and exhaling slowly, drawing your belly back in. The emphasis is on slow, controlled breaths, which stimulate the parasympathetic nervous system, responsible for the "rest and digest" response, counteracting the effects of the stress response. Various breathing exercises, such as box breathing (inhaling for four counts, holding for four, exhaling for four, and holding for four) or alternate nostril breathing (Nadi Shodhana), can be easily learned and incorporated into daily life. These techniques are particularly helpful in managing immediate stress responses, such as before a presentation or during a challenging situation. Regular practice of deep breathing can even improve cardiovascular health and reduce blood pressure, further enhancing overall well-being.

Spending time in
nature
offers a remarkable antidote to stress. Studies have shown that even brief exposure to
natural environments can lower cortisol levels and reduce feelings of anxiety and depression. Whether it's a walk in the park, a hike in the woods, or simply sitting by a lake, connecting with nature offers a restorative effect. The sights, sounds, and smells of nature can promote relaxation and provide a sense of peace and tranquility. Natural environments offer a break from the constant stimulation of urban life, allowing your mind to rest and recharge. This doesn't necessarily require elaborate excursions; even a short walk in your neighborhood park or tending to plants in your garden can provide therapeutic benefits. Engaging with nature fosters a sense of calm, enhances creativity, and allows for a mindful disconnection from the stressors of daily life.

Social support
is also a crucial component of stress
management. Connecting with friends, family, or support groups provides a sense of belonging and shared experience, easing the burden of stress. Sharing your feelings and concerns with trusted individuals can provide emotional support and validation, helping to process difficult emotions and gain valuable perspective. Strong social connections have been linked to improved mental and physical health outcomes, reducing the negative impact of stress. It's crucial to build and maintain positive relationships, fostering open communication and mutual support. This may involve actively making time for social interactions, engaging in shared activities, or simply making time for meaningful conversations. The simple act of connecting with another human being can create a powerful sense of emotional connection, easing the isolation and anxiety often associated with stress.

In addition to these techniques, incorporating
**regular
physical activity**
is a potent stress reliever. Exercise releases endorphins, which have mood-boosting and pain-relieving effects. This doesn't necessarily mean intense workouts; even moderate exercise, such as a brisk walk or a gentle swim, can have positive effects on stress levels. Finding an enjoyable activity – whether it's dancing, cycling, hiking, or strength training – increases the likelihood of sticking with it. The key is consistency and choosing activities that you genuinely enjoy. The benefits of exercise extend far beyond stress reduction; it also contributes to weight management, improves sleep, and boosts overall physical health, creating a positive feedback loop that reinforces your healthy lifestyle choices.

Time management techniques
can greatly reduce stress related to work, family, and other obligations. Prioritizing tasks, setting realistic goals, and learning to say no to non-essential commitments can significantly reduce feelings of overwhelm and anxiety. Utilizing tools like planners, to-do lists, or time-blocking techniques can help you manage your time more effectively. Breaking down large tasks into
smaller, more manageable steps can also make them feel less daunting. The goal is to cultivate a sense of control over your time and commitments, reducing feelings of being overwhelmed or out of control. By strategically allocating your time and focusing on what truly matters, you can mitigate the stress associated with juggling multiple responsibilities.

Cognitive restructuring
is a therapeutic technique that involves identifying and challenging negative or irrational thoughts that contribute to stress. This process involves learning to reframe negative thoughts into more realistic and positive ones. For instance, instead of thinking "I'll never succeed," you might reframe this as "This is challenging, but

I can learn and grow from this experience." Cognitive restructuring requires self-awareness and practice, but it can be a powerful tool for managing stress and improving overall mental well-being. Working with a therapist or counselor can provide guidance and support in developing this skill. This approach helps to manage stress by addressing the root cause– negative thinking patterns – providing a long-term solution for managing stress effectively.

Finally, ensuring adequate
nutritional intake
is integral to stress management. The Carnivore and Paleo diets, with their emphasis on whole, unprocessed foods, provide
essential nutrients that support overall health and well-being. A balanced diet, rich in protein, healthy fats, and essential vitamins and minerals, is crucial for maintaining hormonal balance, energy levels, and resilience to stress. Paying attention to nutrient deficiencies and addressing them through dietary adjustments or supplementation can significantly improve your ability to manage stress effectively. Adequate hydration is also critical, as dehydration can exacerbate feelings of stress and anxiety. By focusing on a nutrient-dense diet, you are equipping your body with the tools it needs to cope with stress effectively and maintain optimal functioning. This holistic approach underscores the interconnectedness of diet, stress, and overall well-being, emphasizing that supporting your body nutritionally is an important aspect of managing stress levels effectively. Remember, sustainable weight loss and lasting well-being are built upon a foundation of holistic self-care, where stress management is not an optional add-on, but a crucial element that intertwines seamlessly with diet, exercise, and sleep.

Integrating Stress Management into Daily Life

Building upon the foundation of nutritional adequacy discussed earlier, let's delve into practical strategies for integrating stress management into your daily routine. Remember, the goal isn't to eliminate stress entirely—that's unrealistic—but to develop resilience and coping mechanisms that allow you to navigate stressful situations without derailing your weight loss progress or overall well-being. The Carnivore and Paleo diets provide a solid nutritional base, but their success is amplified when paired with effective stress management techniques.

One highly effective technique is mindfulness meditation. Even just five to ten minutes a day of focused attention on your breath, body sensations, or a guided meditation can significantly reduce stress hormones and improve your overall sense of calm. Numerous apps offer guided meditations for beginners, making it easily accessible. Start with short sessions and gradually increase the duration as you become more comfortable. The key is consistency; even a few minutes each day will yield better results than sporadic longer sessions.

Another readily accessible tool is deep breathing exercises. These simple techniques can be practiced anywhere, anytime, and require no special equipment. The 4-7-8 breathing technique, for example, involves inhaling deeply for a count of four, holding your breath for seven, and exhaling slowly for eight. Repeating this several times can quickly calm your nervous system and reduce feelings of anxiety. Similar techniques, such as box breathing (equal counts for inhale, hold, exhale, and hold), can be equally effective and easily adapted to your preference.

Regular physical activity, beyond the structured exercise mentioned previously, also plays a crucial role in stress reduction. A brisk walk in nature, a yoga session, or even a short burst of high-intensity interval training (HIIT) can release endorphins, natural mood boosters that combat stress and improve overall mood. Choose activities you genuinely enjoy, as this enhances adherence and makes exercise a less of a chore and more of a stress-relieving activity. The key is to find movement that feels restorative, rather than adding another source of pressure to your schedule.

Prioritizing social connections is also vital. Spending time with loved ones, engaging in meaningful conversations, and cultivating supportive relationships can significantly buffer against stress. Humans are social creatures, and strong social bonds provide a sense of belonging and security, reducing feelings of isolation and loneliness, both of which can exacerbate stress. This could involve scheduling regular phone calls with family or friends, joining a local club or group based on your interests, or simply making time for quality conversations with those close to you.

Incorporating enjoyable hobbies and activities into your daily routine is equally important. Engaging in activities you find pleasurable helps to shift your focus away from stressors and fosters a sense of relaxation and rejuvenation. This might involve reading, listening to music, gardening, painting, or any other activity that brings you joy and a sense of accomplishment. These activities aren't simply distractions; they actively contribute to stress reduction by promoting a sense of well-being and helping you maintain a balanced lifestyle.

Beyond these direct stress-reduction techniques, consider incorporating elements that foster a more relaxed and calming environment. This could involve creating a dedicated relaxation space in your home, a quiet corner where you can retreat to unwind and de-stress. Consider incorporating elements that promote relaxation, such as soft lighting, calming music, comfortable seating, and perhaps even aromatherapy. This personal sanctuary provides a space to escape the pressures of daily life and recharge your batteries.

Sleep hygiene, as discussed previously, is directly connected to stress management. Lack of sleep exacerbates stress, impairing your ability to cope with challenging situations. Prioritizing consistent sleep patterns, maintaining a regular sleep schedule, creating a conducive sleep environment (dark, quiet, cool), and engaging in relaxing bedtime routines significantly improves sleep quality. Avoiding caffeine and alcohol before bed, ensuring adequate hydration, and engaging in relaxing activities like reading or taking a warm bath can all contribute to improved sleep, indirectly managing stress levels.

Journaling can also be a powerful tool for stress management. Regularly writing down your thoughts and feelings, particularly any anxieties or stressors, can help to process emotions, gain clarity, and reduce the mental burden of unresolved issues. It's a way to externalize internal pressures, giving you a sense of control and perspective. You don't need to write eloquently; the simple act of putting your feelings down on paper can be incredibly therapeutic.

Time management is another essential aspect of stress reduction. Effective time management strategies help prevent feeling overwhelmed, which is a major contributor to stress. Prioritize tasks, break down large projects into smaller, more manageable steps, and learn to delegate where possible. Utilize tools like planners or apps to organize your schedule and stay on track. The sense of control gained from effectively managing your time contributes significantly to reduced stress and improved overall well-being.

Finally, consider seeking professional support if stress is significantly impacting your life. A therapist or counselor can provide guidance and support in developing coping mechanisms and strategies for managing stress effectively. They can offer evidence-based techniques such as Cognitive Behavioral Therapy (CBT), which helps identify and modify negative thought patterns and behaviors that contribute to stress. Don't hesitate to reach out for professional help if you feel overwhelmed or unable to manage your stress effectively on your own. It's a sign of strength, not weakness, to seek support when needed.

Integrating these stress-management techniques into your daily life is a process, not a destination. Start by incorporating one or two techniques that resonate with you, and gradually add others as you become more comfortable. Remember, consistency is key. Even small, consistent efforts will yield significant improvements in your ability to manage stress, boosting your overall well-being and enhancing the success of your weight loss journey. The interconnectedness of diet, exercise, sleep, and stress management cannot be overstated; they form the pillars of a holistic and sustainable approach to weight management and a healthier lifestyle. By nurturing each aspect, you are not only achieving your weight goals but also fostering a resilient and balanced self, equipped to navigate life's challenges with grace and ease. The ultimate goal is not just weight loss, but lasting well-being, achieved through a holistic and sustainable approach. Remember to celebrate small victories and be patient with yourself throughout this journey. The path to a healthier and happier you is paved with consistent effort and self-compassion.

Dealing with Food Cravings

Food cravings are a common challenge for anyone embarking on a weight loss journey, and the Carnivore-Paleo approach is no exception. Understanding and managing these cravings is crucial for long-term success. The key is to address the underlying causes and develop effective coping strategies rather than simply suppressing them with willpower alone. Let's explore a multifaceted approach to conquering those tempting cravings.

First, it's important to understand
why
you're experiencing cravings. Often, cravings aren't simply about a desire for a specific food; they're signals from your body indicating an underlying need. These needs might include insufficient nutrients, dehydration, lack of sleep, stress, or even
hormonal imbalances. Keeping a food journal can be incredibly helpful in identifying patterns and triggers. Note down what you ate, when you ate it, how you felt before and after eating, and the specific cravings you experienced. Over time, this journal will reveal connections between your cravings and various factors in your life. For example, you might discover that your sugar cravings always surface after a particularly stressful day at work or that your late-night cravings are linked to insufficient protein intake earlier in the day.

Once you've identified your triggers, you can begin to address them proactively. If dehydration is a culprit, ensure you're consistently drinking enough water throughout the day. Consider carrying a water bottle with you and setting reminders on your phone. If stress is a major factor, incorporate stress-reducing techniques into your daily routine. This could include meditation, yoga, deep breathing exercises, spending time in nature, or engaging in hobbies you enjoy. Prioritizing sufficient sleep is also vital, as sleep deprivation can disrupt hormones that regulate appetite and increase cravings. Aim for 7-9 hours of quality sleep each night by establishing a consistent sleep schedule and creating a relaxing bedtime routine.

Nutritional deficiencies can also fuel cravings. While the Carnivore-Paleo diet focuses on whole, nutrient-dense foods, it's still possible to experience deficiencies, especially if your diet lacks variety. For example, a lack of vitamin C can lead to cravings for sugary foods. If you suspect a nutrient deficiency, consult with a healthcare professional or registered dietitian to determine if supplementation is necessary. They can help you identify potential deficiencies through blood tests and recommend appropriate supplements to address them.

Beyond addressing underlying causes, you can also employ strategies to manage cravings directly. One effective technique is
mindful eating
. Before you give in to a
craving, take a moment to pause and ask yourself if you're truly hungry or if the craving is driven by emotion, stress, or habit. Pay attention to your body's hunger cues. Are you genuinely experiencing physical hunger pangs, or is it merely a mental desire for a specific food? If it's the latter, try engaging in a distracting activity such as taking a walk, reading a book, or calling a friend. This can often help you to shift your focus away from the craving.

Another strategy involves finding healthy substitutes that satisfy your cravings without compromising your dietary goals. If you crave the sweetness of fruit, try berries or a small amount of honey. If you're craving the crunch of chips, try celery sticks with guacamole or a handful of macadamia nuts. Remember that the goal is not to eliminate cravings entirely; it's to find healthy alternatives that satisfy your needs without sabotaging your progress.

For those experiencing intense cravings, it can be helpful to gradually introduce small amounts of the craved food in a controlled manner. This can help to reduce the intensity of the craving over time. For example, if you crave bread, start with a small slice of sourdough bread, noting how it makes you feel. This controlled exposure can help to break the cycle of intense craving and eventual overindulgence. However, this approach should be done cautiously and in consultation with a healthcare professional, especially when considering reintroducing carbohydrates.

It's also important to emphasize the importance of self-compassion. Everyone experiences setbacks, and it's crucial to avoid harsh self-criticism when cravings get the better of you. Instead of dwelling on the indulgence, acknowledge it, learn from the experience, and refocus on your overall goals. A single slip-up does not negate all the hard work you've put in.

Remember, managing food cravings is a process, not a destination. It takes time, patience, and self-awareness to develop effective coping strategies. By identifying your triggers, addressing underlying needs, practicing mindful eating, and finding healthy substitutes, you can learn to navigate cravings effectively and stay on track with your Carnivore-Paleo journey. Remember that seeking professional guidance from a registered dietitian or healthcare provider can be incredibly beneficial in personalizing strategies and addressing specific concerns. They can offer personalized advice and support, helping you to develop a sustainable and effective plan that works for you. Don't hesitate to reach out for help when needed—it's a sign of strength, not weakness. With persistence and a holistic approach, you can overcome food cravings and achieve sustainable weight loss.

Furthermore, consider the emotional aspects of food cravings. Often, cravings are linked to emotional states like stress, boredom, or sadness. When a craving hits, take a moment to check in with your emotions. Are you feeling overwhelmed, anxious, or lonely? If so, address the underlying emotional issue rather than reaching for food as a temporary fix. Engage in activities that soothe and comfort you, such as spending time with loved ones, listening to music, or taking a warm bath.

Finally, remember the importance of planning ahead, especially for social events and holidays. These occasions can present unique challenges, as tempting foods are often abundant. Before attending a gathering, have a plan in place. Decide in advance what you'll eat and how much you'll consume. Bring a healthy alternative with you if needed, and don't be afraid to politely decline unwanted dishes. By preparing for potential pitfalls, you can reduce the likelihood of impulsive eating and maintain your dietary goals. Remember, long-term success relies on consistency and a sustainable approach; don't be discouraged by occasional challenges. With planning, self-compassion, and mindful strategies, you can successfully manage food cravings and achieve your health and wellness objectives. This is a journey, not a race, so embrace the process and celebrate your progress along the way.

Navigating Social Gatherings and Holidays

Social events and holidays often present unique challenges to anyone following a dietary plan, and the Carnivore-Paleo approach is no exception. The abundance of tempting, often carb-heavy and processed foods can make staying on track feel nearly impossible. However, with careful planning and a proactive mindset, you can navigate these situations with grace and maintain your commitment to a healthy lifestyle. The key is to view these events not as obstacles, but as opportunities to practice your self-control and demonstrate your dedication to your wellness goals.

First, let's address the planning aspect. Before attending any social gathering or holiday celebration, take some time to mentally prepare. Review the planned menu if it's available. Identify potential pitfalls – high-carbohydrate dishes, sugary desserts, or processed snacks. Knowing what challenges you might encounter empowers you to make informed decisions beforehand. This preemptive planning reduces the likelihood of making impulsive choices in the heat of the moment when willpower is often weakest.

One powerful strategy is to eat a satisfying Carnivore-Paleo meal beforehand. This pre-emptive measure prevents you from arriving ravenous and susceptible to overeating less healthy options. A well-balanced meal consisting of quality protein, healthy fats, and perhaps some low-carb vegetables will keep your blood sugar stable and reduce cravings for less-suitable foods. Think a hearty steak, some grilled salmon, or a delicious bone broth with some added collagen. This satiety strategy ensures you aren't easily tempted by less-ideal food choices at the event itself.

Next, consider bringing a safe and delicious alternative. Pack a small, easily portable snack or appetizer that aligns with your Carnivore-Paleo principles. This could be a piece of leftover steak, some hard-boiled eggs, a small container of macadamia nuts (if you include nuts in your variation of the diet), or even some cheese sticks. Having a backup plan helps avoid feeling deprived and enables you to participate in the social event without compromising your dietary goals. It's a powerful tool to prevent hunger-driven choices that could derail your progress.

Remember the importance of mindful eating. At social gatherings, pay attention to your body's hunger and fullness cues. Avoid mindless eating; put your fork down between bites and savor each mouthful. This conscious approach prevents overeating even of permissible foods. Take your time, engage in conversation, and focus on the company, not just the food. This mindful approach significantly increases your enjoyment of the social interaction while simultaneously controlling your intake.

When faced with tempting, non-compliant foods, practice polite refusal. You don't need to make excuses or elaborate on your dietary choices. A simple, "No thank you, I'm good," is perfectly acceptable. Focus on enjoying the company and the overall atmosphere of the event. Remember that your health journey is personal, and you don't need to justify your choices to anyone else. Confidently navigating these social situations reinforces your commitment to your well-being. Your dedication to your health choices should be a source of pride, not a source of self-consciousness.

Navigating holiday gatherings requires similar strategies, albeit often on a larger scale. Holidays often involve a wide array of tempting dishes, extended family gatherings, and the added pressure of social expectations. Plan your approach with even more careful consideration. Before the festivities, communicate with your hosts. This doesn't mean you need to impose your dietary restrictions, but simply letting them know you're following a specific eating plan will often prompt them to offer a compatible option. Many hosts appreciate knowing your preferences beforehand and are often willing to accommodate them.

For larger holiday meals, focus on the items that align with your Carnivore-Paleo principles. Fill your plate with those dishes, and take only small portions of anything you're unsure about. It's perfectly acceptable to taste a small amount of a tempting dish, but remember that moderation is key. The goal isn't to completely eliminate enjoyment of holiday treats, but rather to consume them mindfully and in moderation, without feeling guilty or significantly derailing your progress.

If there aren't any suitable options, bring a dish you know you can enjoy. This ensures you have something healthy and satisfying to eat, regardless of what others bring. Perhaps a simple side salad with an olive oil and lemon dressing (if vegetables are part of your chosen dietary variation) or a perfectly cooked piece of meat will make sure you don't leave the event feeling deprived or unsatisfied.

Consider that holiday gatherings often involve more than just food. Focus on connecting with family and friends. Engage in conversations, play games, and participate in the activities. The social aspect of these gatherings is often more rewarding than the food itself. By shifting your attention to the social connection, you'll find that the allure of unhealthy food becomes less of a temptation.

Dealing with potential peer pressure is a crucial aspect of navigating social events while adhering to a specialized diet. Friends and family may not fully understand your dietary choices. They might offer unsolicited advice, express concern, or even try to pressure you into eating things that are not part of your plan. It is crucial to have a prepared response, one that confidently and politely reaffirms your commitment to your health goals.

One effective strategy is to simply explain the core tenets of your diet. For example, you might say: "I'm focusing on a high-protein, low-carbohydrate diet to improve my overall health. I'm feeling much better since making these changes and am committed to maintaining this plan." This concise explanation avoids lengthy justifications and clearly communicates your intentions.

Another helpful approach is to focus on the positive aspects of your dietary choices. Instead of dwelling on what you're avoiding, highlight the benefits you're experiencing. For instance, you could say, "I've noticed a significant increase in my energy levels since changing my diet. I feel so much better!" This emphasizes the positive outcomes of your lifestyle change, making your choices more understandable and less subject to criticism.

If someone persistently tries to pressure you to eat something that is against your dietary principles, a firm yet polite "No, thank you" is perfectly acceptable. You don't owe anyone an explanation beyond that. Remember, your health and well-being are your responsibility, and it's perfectly acceptable to prioritize those needs.

While adhering to the Carnivore-Paleo approach during social events and holidays requires planning and self-discipline, it's definitely achievable. It's about finding a balance between enjoying social occasions and staying true to your dietary goals. By implementing these strategies—planning ahead, bringing healthy alternatives, practicing mindful eating, politely declining unwanted items, and focusing on the social aspects of the gathering—you can successfully navigate these situations without compromising your commitment to a healthy and sustainable lifestyle. Remember, this journey is about making long-term changes for sustained well-being. Don't let a few social gatherings derail your progress. Celebrate your successes, learn from minor setbacks, and focus on the long-term benefits of your healthy choices. Your success is entirely within your reach.

Managing Plateaus and Maintaining Motivation

Weight loss isn't always a linear journey. You might experience periods where the scale stubbornly refuses to budge, despite your diligent adherence to the Carnivore-Paleo principles. These frustrating periods, known as weight loss plateaus, are perfectly normal and don't signify failure. Instead, they represent a shift in your body's adaptation to your new lifestyle. Your metabolism might be adjusting to the lower calorie intake, or your body might be conserving energy more efficiently. Understanding this process is crucial to overcoming the plateau and maintaining your motivation.

One common cause of plateaus is a slowing metabolism. As you lose weight, your body requires fewer calories to maintain its functions. This is a natural response, and it doesn't mean you're doing anything wrong. To counter this, consider slightly adjusting your caloric intake. A small reduction – perhaps 100-200 calories per day – can reignite the weight loss process. Remember, precise calorie counting isn't necessary on a Carnivore-Paleo diet; focus instead on maintaining satiety and consuming nutrient-dense foods. If a reduction doesn't work, consider increasing your physical activity.

Another factor contributing to plateaus is a lack of sufficient physical activity. While the Carnivore-Paleo diet can naturally boost metabolism and satiety, regular exercise is essential for long-term weight management and overall health. If you've been sticking to the same exercise routine for several weeks, try incorporating variations to challenge your body. This could involve increasing the intensity, duration, or frequency of your workouts. Experiment with different activities to find what you enjoy most. Walking, swimming, strength training, and high-intensity interval training (HIIT) are all excellent choices, but the key is to find something sustainable and enjoyable.

Beyond physical changes, plateaus can be profoundly impacted by psychological factors. Motivation is a crucial component of successful weight loss. When progress slows, it's easy to feel discouraged and lose steam. Maintaining motivation requires a proactive approach. Begin by re-evaluating your goals. Are they still realistic and relevant? If your goals seem daunting or unattainable, break them down into smaller, more manageable steps. This approach fosters a sense of accomplishment and keeps you motivated. Regularly celebrate small victories, no matter how insignificant they might seem. This positive reinforcement keeps you focused on the progress you've already made and encourages you to continue.

Tracking your progress is an essential strategy to maintain momentum during weight loss plateaus. Regularly weigh yourself, but don't focus solely on the number on the scale. Pay attention to other indicators of progress, such as improvements in energy levels, sleep quality, and fitness performance. Take progress photos to visually track changes in body composition. These alternative measures provide a broader perspective and can be incredibly motivating when the scale seems stuck. Remember that weight loss is only one aspect of overall health and well-being. Focusing solely on the number on the scale can lead to disappointment and discouragement, especially during plateaus.

Another powerful motivational tool is the support system. Surrounding yourself with a supportive community can significantly improve your chances of overcoming weight loss plateaus. This could involve joining online forums or groups dedicated to the Carnivore-Paleo diet, finding a weight loss buddy, or seeking support from family and friends. Sharing your experiences, challenges, and victories can reinforce your commitment and help you stay accountable. A support system offers encouragement and understanding, especially during challenging times. Don't hesitate to reach out to others for help; many people have encountered similar challenges and can offer valuable advice and encouragement.

Stress management is yet another crucial aspect of navigating plateaus and sustaining motivation. Chronic stress can disrupt hormones related to appetite and metabolism, potentially leading to weight gain or hindering weight loss. Incorporate stress-reducing activities into your daily routine, such as meditation, yoga, deep breathing exercises, or spending time in nature. Prioritize sufficient sleep, as lack of sleep can also negatively impact hormones and increase appetite. Aim for seven to nine hours of quality sleep per night. Adequate sleep is essential for physical and mental well-being and significantly contributes to successful weight loss.

Finally, remember that setbacks are inevitable. Don't let occasional slip-ups derail your progress. Instead, view them as learning opportunities. Analyze what triggered the setback and adjust your plan accordingly. Perhaps you need to refine your meal preparation strategies, improve your stress management techniques, or seek additional support. Don't be afraid to ask for professional guidance. A registered dietitian or nutritionist specializing in low-carbohydrate diets can provide personalized advice and support to help you overcome challenges and maintain motivation. Remember, weight loss is a marathon, not a sprint. Progress isn't always linear; there will be ups and downs along the way. Embrace the journey, focus on your overall well-being, and celebrate your successes.

Plateaus often involve a reassessment of your dietary habits. Have you been consistently tracking your food intake, even though calorie counting isn't a strict requirement on Carnivore-Paleo? A food diary can reveal hidden patterns or inconsistencies. Are you consuming enough electrolytes? Electrolyte imbalances are common on low-carbohydrate diets and can cause fatigue, muscle cramps, and water retention, potentially masking true weight loss. Ensure adequate intake of sodium, potassium, and magnesium.

Consider exploring variations within the Carnivore-Paleo framework. If you've been strictly Carnivore, consider incorporating a wider range of animal products, or selectively adding nutrient-dense vegetables. If you're already incorporating vegetables, consider focusing on higher nutrient density options like leafy greens or cruciferous vegetables, ensuring they don't negatively impact satiety. However, be mindful of potential impacts on gut health and adjust your intake slowly to avoid digestive discomfort. Remember, the Carnivore-Paleo approach is about finding the optimal balance for your individual needs and preferences.

Addressing potential hormonal imbalances is also essential. Conditions like hypothyroidism can significantly impact metabolism and weight management. If you suspect a hormonal imbalance, it's crucial to seek medical evaluation and appropriate treatment from a qualified healthcare professional. Addressing underlying hormonal issues can play a significant role in overcoming weight loss plateaus and achieving your weight management goals.

Let's not overlook the importance of mindful eating. Are you eating slowly and paying attention to your hunger and fullness cues? Mindful eating helps you connect with your body's signals, preventing overeating. Are you eating in a relaxed environment, free from distractions? Distracted eating can lead to increased calorie consumption without conscious awareness. Consider the timing of your meals and snacks. Are you consuming food at regular intervals? Irregular eating patterns can disrupt your metabolism and hinder weight loss.

Beyond the practical dietary aspects, consider the influence of sleep deprivation. Insufficient sleep can disrupt hormones that regulate appetite and metabolism, leading to increased hunger and cravings. Aim for seven to nine hours of quality sleep each night. Establish a consistent sleep schedule, create a relaxing bedtime routine, and optimize your sleep environment for a restful night's sleep. The improvement in your overall well-being alone may provide significant motivational benefits.

Finally, remember that weight loss is a holistic process. While the Carnivore-Paleo approach is a powerful tool, it's only one piece of the puzzle. Addressing emotional well-being, stress management, and building a strong support system are essential for long-term success. Celebrate your achievements along the way, and remember that every small step forward contributes to your overall progress. Persistence and a positive mindset are key to overcoming plateaus and maintaining the momentum needed to reach your weight management goals. The journey may have its challenges, but the rewards of a healthier, more vibrant life are well worth the effort.

Addressing Potential Nutrient Deficiencies

While the Carnivore-Paleo approach emphasizes whole, nutrient-dense foods, it's crucial to be mindful of potential nutrient deficiencies. Restricting food groups, even intentionally, can lead to imbalances if not carefully managed. This section will address common concerns and provide practical strategies for ensuring you obtain all the nutrients your body needs to thrive.

One of the primary concerns with highly restrictive diets is the potential for vitamin deficiencies. Fruits and vegetables, often limited on the Carnivore-Paleo diet, are rich sources of vitamins A, C, and various B vitamins. A deficiency in Vitamin C, for example, can lead to scurvy, characterized by fatigue, weakness, and bleeding gums. Vitamin A deficiency can impact vision and immune function. B vitamin deficiencies can manifest as fatigue, anemia, and neurological problems. To mitigate these risks, careful consideration of nutrient intake is paramount.

While a purely carnivorous approach may seem straightforward, ensuring adequate vitamin intake requires proactive measures. Supplementation may be necessary, particularly Vitamin C, which is readily available in inexpensive and effective supplements. For Vitamin A, it's important to choose sources of animal products that naturally contain this vitamin. Organ meats, such as liver, are exceptionally rich in Vitamin A. Including small amounts of nutrient-dense vegetables, such as leafy greens or cruciferous vegetables, can also contribute significantly to vitamin intake without compromising the core principles of the diet.

Mineral deficiencies are another potential issue. Minerals such as magnesium, potassium, and zinc play vital roles in various bodily functions. Magnesium is essential for muscle function, nerve transmission, and blood sugar control. Potassium is critical for maintaining healthy blood pressure and fluid balance. Zinc is crucial for immune function, wound healing, and cell growth. These minerals are abundant in many plant-based foods, including leafy greens, nuts, and seeds. The restricted nature of the Carnivore-Paleo approach can lead to insufficient intake, especially if plant-based foods are significantly limited.

To address potential mineral deficiencies, strategic supplementation may be beneficial. For magnesium, supplementation can easily address any deficiency. Potassium supplements are also available, but it's crucial to consult with a healthcare professional before starting supplementation, as excessive potassium can be harmful. Paying attention to the mineral content of the animal products consumed is also essential. Grass-fed animals, for instance, generally have higher levels of certain minerals compared to grain-fed counterparts.

Fiber intake is another significant consideration. Fiber, primarily found in plant-based foods, plays a crucial role in digestive health, promoting regularity and preventing constipation. Low fiber intake can also lead to issues with blood sugar control. While the absence of fiber isn't immediately life-threatening in the short term, its long-term absence can have serious negative consequences on digestive health and general well-being. Addressing this requires careful planning and consideration.

If adopting a very strict Carnivore diet, where virtually all plant matter is excluded, addressing the fiber deficit becomes crucial. Psyllium husk, a fiber supplement derived from the seeds of the Plantago ovata plant, offers a viable solution without significantly deviating from the core principles of the Carnivore-Paleo approach. It's important to note, though, that incorporating psyllium husk requires gradual introduction to avoid digestive upset. Always begin with a small dose and gradually increase it over time as tolerated.

Beyond vitamins, minerals, and fiber, the issue of fatty acid balance should also be considered. Omega-3 fatty acids, crucial for brain health, heart health, and reducing inflammation, are more abundant in fatty fish. However, ensuring a balanced intake of omega-3s and omega-6s is essential. An over-reliance on red meat might skew this balance, potentially increasing the risk of inflammation.

Addressing this necessitates mindful selection of protein sources. Incorporating fatty fish like salmon, mackerel, and sardines regularly can help maintain a healthy omega-3 to omega-6 ratio. While some advocate for consuming organ meats for their concentrated nutrients, excessive consumption of organ meats can lead to an overconsumption of certain vitamins and minerals such as Vitamin A. Therefore, moderation is always key. Listening to your body's signals and adjusting your intake accordingly is of paramount importance.

The potential for nutrient deficiencies on the Carnivore-Paleo diet highlights the importance of careful planning and monitoring. Regular blood tests to monitor vitamin and mineral levels are recommended, particularly in the initial stages of the diet. These tests provide valuable insights into your nutritional status, allowing for adjustments in your diet or supplementation strategy as needed.

Many individuals successfully follow the Carnivore-Paleo approach without experiencing significant nutrient deficiencies. However, understanding the potential risks and implementing preventative strategies is crucial for long-term health and well-being. Prioritizing whole, nutrient-dense animal products, mindful supplementation where necessary, and regular blood testing are all essential elements for navigating the potential challenges and maximizing the benefits of this dietary approach.

Regular blood tests should be performed at least annually to monitor your vitamin and mineral levels. These tests provide invaluable data that allow you to identify any deficiencies before they manifest as symptoms. Your healthcare provider can guide you on the specific tests required and interpret the results. They can also provide personalized recommendations for supplementation if necessary.

Beyond laboratory testing, paying close attention to your body's signals is equally important. Persistent fatigue, weakness, hair loss, skin problems, or digestive issues could all indicate underlying nutritional deficiencies. If you experience any of these symptoms, don't hesitate to seek guidance from a healthcare professional or registered dietitian. They can help you identify potential deficiencies and develop a plan to address them.

Remember that the Carnivore-Paleo approach is not a one-size-fits-all solution. Individual nutritional needs vary, and what works for one person might not work for another.
Listening to your body and adapting your dietary choices accordingly is crucial for achieving optimal health and well-being on this or any dietary approach. The information provided in this chapter is intended for educational purposes and should not be considered medical advice. Always consult with a healthcare professional before making significant dietary changes, particularly if you have any

underlying health conditions. They can help you assess your individual needs and develop a safe and effective plan.

This careful and proactive approach ensures that while adhering to the principles of the Carnivore-Paleo diet, you are minimizing the risks associated with nutrient deficiencies and maximizing the benefits for your long-term health. The key lies in balance, careful planning, and consistent monitoring – a holistic approach that ensures the diet's success not just in terms of weight loss but also overall well-being. Don't be afraid to seek professional guidance; it can make all the difference in your journey towards a healthier lifestyle. Remember, the goal is to nourish your body while achieving your weight management goals, not to compromise your health in the process.

Seeking Professional Guidance

Embarking on any significant dietary change, especially one as focused as the Carnivore-Paleo approach, requires a thoughtful and individualized strategy. While this book provides a comprehensive framework, recognizing your limitations and seeking professional guidance when necessary is crucial. This isn't a sign of weakness; it's a testament to your commitment to achieving sustainable, healthy weight loss. Many individuals thrive independently, but others benefit significantly from personalized support.

Let's explore scenarios where seeking professional help is particularly beneficial. First and foremost, if you have any pre-existing health conditions, such as diabetes, kidney disease, heart conditions, autoimmune disorders, or gastrointestinal issues, consulting your physician or a registered dietitian (RD) is non-negotiable
before
starting the Carnivore-Paleo diet. These conditions often require careful dietary management, and this approach, with its significant restrictions, might necessitate modifications or contraindications. Your doctor can assess your overall health, identify potential risks, and help you tailor the diet to your specific needs, ensuring it aligns with your medical profile and doesn't exacerbate any existing problems. They can also monitor your progress and make necessary adjustments to your treatment plan if needed. An RD can provide detailed guidance on nutrient intake, ensuring you're meeting your daily requirements and avoiding potential deficiencies.

Secondly, if you're experiencing unexpected or concerning side effects, don't hesitate to reach out for professional medical attention. While some initial adjustments are normal—such as changes in bowel habits or energy levels—

persistent or severe symptoms like headaches, dizziness, nausea, fatigue, or unexplained weight loss require immediate medical evaluation. These could indicate underlying health issues that need prompt diagnosis and treatment. Delaying medical attention in such instances can be detrimental to your health. Remember, the goal is to improve your well-being, not jeopardize it.

Furthermore, consider seeking professional guidance if you struggle to maintain the diet consistently or encounter unexpected hurdles. Weight loss is a journey, not a race, and everyone encounters challenges. An RD or a health coach can provide personalized support, helping you overcome plateaus, address emotional eating patterns, or navigate social situations where adhering to the diet might be difficult. They can offer practical strategies for meal planning, grocery shopping, and managing cravings. They can also provide coping mechanisms for dealing with social pressures related to food, assisting you in maintaining a positive and sustainable approach to your health journey. Remember, consistent support can often make the difference between success and failure.

The role of a registered dietitian extends beyond simply creating meal plans. They can perform comprehensive nutritional assessments, analyzing your current diet, identifying potential deficiencies, and recommending strategies to address them. This assessment may involve blood tests to measure nutrient levels and assess overall health markers. They can help you create a personalized plan that addresses your unique nutritional needs, ensuring you're not sacrificing essential vitamins and minerals for weight loss. They can also educate you about the importance of nutrient timing and the role of various macronutrients in your body. Moreover, they can adapt the Carnivore-Paleo principles to meet your specific dietary requirements and preferences, offering a more manageable and sustainable approach.

For individuals with specific dietary needs or allergies, professional guidance is especially valuable. For example, if you have food allergies or intolerances, an RD can help you carefully select foods to avoid triggering reactions, ensuring the diet remains safe and effective for you. They can help you navigate potential cross-contamination issues and identify suitable alternatives. Similarly, individuals with specific nutrient requirements, such as pregnant or breastfeeding women, or those with specific metabolic conditions, should consult with a healthcare professional before making any significant dietary changes. The Carnivore-Paleo diet, while beneficial for many, might not be suitable for everyone, and professional guidance ensures you make informed choices that support your health.

Beyond the medical aspects, seeking professional support can also address the psychological and emotional aspects of weight loss. Many individuals struggle with emotional eating or have ingrained habits that make healthy eating challenging. A registered dietitian or a health and wellness coach can help identify these patterns and develop strategies to overcome them. This could involve cognitive behavioral therapy (CBT) techniques or other behavioral modification strategies to help you manage cravings, stress, and emotional triggers that might lead to unhealthy eating habits. Support groups and online communities are useful resources, providing peer support and encouragement. However, professional guidance provides a structured approach tailored to your individual needs.

Furthermore, the long-term maintenance of weight loss is a crucial aspect often overlooked. Many people lose weight successfully but then regain it once they stop following a specific diet. Professional guidance can help you develop sustainable lifestyle changes that support long-term weight management and overall wellness. This includes creating balanced meal plans that you can maintain in the long run, integrating regular physical activity into your routine, and developing strategies to manage stress and emotional eating patterns that might lead to weight gain. A professional can help you establish healthy eating habits and exercise routines that fit your lifestyle and preferences, leading to long-term adherence and sustained success. They can also offer strategies for dealing with setbacks or plateaus, ensuring that you stay on track and committed to your goals.

Finally, don't underestimate the value of regular monitoring and progress assessment. A registered dietitian or health professional can track your progress regularly, adjusting your plan as needed. They can monitor your weight, nutrient levels, and overall health markers to ensure the diet is safe and effective for you. This ongoing support fosters a sense of accountability and motivation, helping you stay committed to your goals, providing guidance, encouragement, and adjustments throughout the process. Regular check-ins can identify potential problems early on, preventing them from escalating into major setbacks.

In summary, while the Carnivore-Paleo approach offers a straightforward and potentially effective path to weight loss, it's not a one-size-fits-all solution. Seeking professional guidance from your physician and a registered dietitian, especially when dealing with pre-existing conditions, experiencing unexpected side effects, struggling with adherence, or needing tailored support for specific needs, significantly increases your chances of success and ensures you prioritize your health throughout your weight loss journey. Remember, a collaborative approach combining self-discipline, informed decision-making, and professional support is the key to long-term success and sustainable health. The ultimate goal is not just weight loss but a healthier, more vibrant you.

Transitioning to Maintenance

Transitioning from the weight-loss phase to the maintenance phase requires a shift in mindset and approach. While the initial focus was on creating a significant calorie deficit to shed pounds, the maintenance phase prioritizes sustaining your healthy weight through balanced habits and mindful choices. This isn't about reverting to old eating patterns; rather, it's about integrating the principles you've learned into a long-term lifestyle. The good news is that many of the strategies you've already mastered during your weight loss journey will continue to serve you well during this phase.

The first step involves gradually increasing your caloric intake. This increase shouldn't be drastic; aim for a slow and steady approach. A rapid increase could easily lead to weight regain. Instead of focusing solely on numbers, pay close attention to your hunger cues. Are you feeling satisfied after your meals? If not, you might need to slightly increase your portion sizes or incorporate a healthy snack. Remember the principles of the Carnivore-Paleo approach: prioritize nutrient-dense whole foods, focusing on high-quality protein and healthy fats. This will help you feel full and satisfied on a moderate caloric intake.

Monitoring your weight is still important during the maintenance phase, but it shouldn't become an obsession. Weigh yourself once a week or even bi-weekly. This provides a general overview, allowing you to catch any significant fluctuations early. However, don't panic over minor changes; weight naturally fluctuates due to hydration levels, hormonal changes, and even the time of day. Focus on how your clothes fit, your energy levels, and overall well-being – these are more reliable indicators of your health and progress than the number on the scale.

Maintaining a regular exercise routine is crucial for long-term success. While the intensity might decrease slightly compared to the weight loss phase, consistency is key. Find activities you enjoy – whether it's brisk walking, strength training, swimming, or cycling. Remember that physical activity isn't just about burning calories; it contributes significantly to overall health, improves mood, and boosts energy levels. Aim for at least 150 minutes of moderate-intensity aerobic activity or 75 minutes of vigorous-intensity activity per week, along with strength training exercises at least twice a week.

Stress management continues to play a vital role in maintaining your weight. High stress levels can lead to increased cortisol production, which can contribute to weight gain and hinder your progress. Continue practicing stress-reduction techniques such as meditation, yoga, deep breathing exercises, or spending time in nature. These methods help regulate your body's response to stress, promoting better sleep, reducing cravings, and improving overall well-being.

Sleep is another critical factor in weight management. Aim for 7-9 hours of quality sleep each night. Sufficient sleep regulates hormones that control appetite and metabolism. Lack of sleep can disrupt these hormones, leading to increased cravings and difficulty managing your weight. Establish a relaxing bedtime routine, ensuring a dark, quiet, and cool sleeping environment.

Social situations and eating out can pose challenges during the maintenance phase. Preparation is crucial. Plan ahead, perhaps by packing a healthy meal or snack to bring along.

When eating out, choose restaurants that align with your dietary preferences. Don't be afraid to ask about ingredients or request modifications to dishes to make them fit your Carnivore-Paleo approach. Remember that occasional indulgences won't derail your progress, as long as they remain just that – occasional.

One of the most critical aspects of successful long-term weight maintenance is developing a flexible approach. Life is unpredictable, and there will be times when your routine is disrupted. Don't let setbacks discourage you; view them as temporary challenges. Adjust your plan as needed, focusing on getting back on track as quickly as possible. Remember that consistent effort, even with minor adjustments, is more effective than perfectionism.

Maintaining your weight loss is a journey, not a destination. It requires ongoing commitment and adaptation. Develop a long-term plan that incorporates the core principles of the Carnivore-Paleo approach, focusing on healthy eating habits, regular exercise, stress management, and sufficient sleep. This will help you create a sustainable lifestyle that promotes both physical and mental well-being. Celebrate your successes along the way; acknowledge your dedication and hard work. Remember the significant changes you've already achieved and continue to build upon this foundation.

Consider developing a detailed meal plan for the maintenance phase. This doesn't have to be as restrictive as your weight-loss meal plan, but it provides a framework to help guide your food choices. Include a variety of protein sources (beef, chicken, fish, eggs), healthy fats (avocado, olive oil, nuts, seeds – depending on your chosen level of adherence), and if including, vegetables. Remember to adjust portion sizes according to your energy needs and hunger cues. Track your meals for a few weeks to ensure you are consuming a balanced and sufficient number of calories.

To maintain motivation, consider setting new, achievable goals. These goals could be related to fitness, such as running a 5k, lifting a certain weight, or completing a particular yoga sequence. Alternatively, focus on non-scale victories, such as increased energy levels, improved sleep, enhanced mood, or better digestion. Celebrate these successes; reward yourself with non-food related rewards, such as a new book, a massage, or a relaxing activity.

Remember to listen to your body. Pay attention to your hunger and fullness cues. Avoid restrictive dieting, as this can lead to nutrient deficiencies and increased cravings.
Instead, cultivate a mindful approach to eating, savoring your meals and being present during your food consumption. This helps you regulate your intake and appreciate your food.

Regular check-ins with a healthcare professional or registered dietitian are beneficial, particularly during the transition to the maintenance phase. They can offer personalized guidance and adjustments to your plan, ensuring you maintain nutritional balance and address any potential concerns. They can monitor your progress, provide support, and help you stay on track.

The maintenance phase is about establishing a sustainable and enjoyable relationship with food and exercise. It's about integrating healthy habits into your daily routine and making them a part of your lifestyle. It requires consistency, flexibility, and a commitment to your well-being. By focusing on these principles and celebrating your achievements, you can successfully maintain your weight loss and enjoy a long and healthy life. Remember that this is a journey, not a race, and there will be ups and downs along the way. The key is to maintain focus on your goals and continue striving for a healthy and sustainable lifestyle. Be proud of your accomplishment and maintain the positive momentum you have built.

Developing a LongTerm Plan

The transition from active weight loss to weight maintenance is not a finish line, but a new starting point—a transition to a lifestyle built on conscious choices that support your health and well-being. This phase demands a shift in perspective. Instead of focusing solely on calorie restriction, the emphasis turns to mindful eating, balanced nutrition, and consistent physical activity. The good news is that many of the strategies you've adopted during weight loss—prioritizing whole, unprocessed foods, managing portion sizes, and staying hydrated—remain crucial for long-term success. However, the rigidity of the initial phase needs to give way to a more flexible, sustainable approach.

One of the most significant adjustments is recalibrating your caloric intake. During weight loss, a significant calorie deficit was essential. In maintenance, however, the goal is to maintain your current weight, requiring a recalculation of your daily energy needs. This involves considering your basal metabolic rate (BMR), activity level, and any other factors influencing your energy expenditure. It's highly recommended to consult a registered dietitian or nutritionist to accurately determine your maintenance calorie needs. This personalized assessment prevents unintentional weight gain or loss while ensuring you receive sufficient nutrients to support your energy levels and overall well-being. Using online calculators can provide an estimate, but professional guidance is invaluable for a precise calculation.

Understanding your body's hunger and fullness cues is paramount. Pay attention to your body's signals; eat when you're truly hungry and stop when you feel comfortably satisfied, not stuffed. This mindful eating approach helps avoid overeating and promotes a healthy relationship with food, reducing the likelihood of emotional eating or impulsive snacking. Regularly checking in with your hunger and fullness cues builds an intuitive understanding of your body's needs, making food choices more deliberate and conscious. It also minimizes the risk of relying on external cues, such as time or social situations, to determine when to eat.

Maintaining regular physical activity is equally crucial. While intense workouts might have been a part of your weight loss strategy, the maintenance phase allows for more flexibility. Focus on activities you genuinely enjoy, whether it's brisk walking, swimming, cycling, weight training, or dancing. The key is consistency rather than intensity. Aim for at least 150 minutes of moderate-intensity aerobic activity or 75 minutes of vigorous-intensity aerobic activity per week, along with muscle-strengthening activities twice a week, as recommended by the U.S. Department of Health and Human Services. However, listen to your body and adjust the intensity and duration based on your fitness level and energy levels. Don't push yourself too hard, especially when starting; gradual progression is key.

Incorporating strength training into your routine is particularly beneficial during weight maintenance. Building muscle mass increases your resting metabolic rate, meaning your body burns more calories even at rest. This helps to prevent weight regain and maintain a healthy body composition. Strength training also offers numerous other benefits, including improved bone density, increased strength and endurance, and enhanced posture. Even simple bodyweight exercises can be effective, especially when combined with consistent effort. Beginners can start with 2-3 sessions per week, gradually increasing the intensity and duration as they gain strength and endurance.

Stress management is often overlooked, but it plays a significant role in weight maintenance. Chronic stress can trigger hormonal imbalances that lead to increased appetite and cravings, often for unhealthy foods. Implementing effective stress-reduction techniques becomes crucial for preventing weight fluctuations. Explore various strategies, such as mindfulness meditation, deep breathing exercises, yoga, spending time in nature, engaging in hobbies, or pursuing social connections. Finding what works best for you is key to ensuring consistent stress management.

Sleep is another often-underestimated aspect of weight maintenance. Adequate sleep supports healthy hormone regulation, reducing the likelihood of increased hunger and cravings. Aim for 7-9 hours of quality sleep per night. Creating a relaxing bedtime routine, ensuring a dark and quiet sleep environment, and avoiding caffeine and alcohol before bed can contribute to better sleep quality. Prioritize sleep alongside nutrition and exercise as a cornerstone of your long-term health plan. Sleep deprivation can negatively impact appetite regulation and increase cortisol levels, potentially leading to weight gain.

Regular monitoring of your weight and body composition is essential, but it shouldn't become an obsession. Weigh yourself once a week, at the same time of day, using the same scale to track any significant changes. However, don't get discouraged by small fluctuations; focus on the overall trend over time. Body composition measurements, such as body fat percentage, can provide a more comprehensive assessment than weight alone, as they reveal changes in muscle mass and fat mass. These measurements can be obtained through professional assessments, such as DEXA scans or bioelectrical impedance analysis.

Celebrate your successes, however small. Acknowledge your achievements and reward yourself with non-food related treats, like a massage, a new book, or a movie night. This positive reinforcement helps maintain your motivation and prevents feelings of deprivation. Remember, maintaining a healthy weight is a journey, not a race, and there will be ups and downs along the way. Don't let occasional setbacks derail your progress. Learn from any challenges and adjust your approach as needed, maintaining a focus on long-term health and well-being.

Building a support system is invaluable. Sharing your journey with friends, family, or a support group provides encouragement and accountability. Consider joining online forums or weight-loss groups for support and inspiration.
Surrounding yourself with positive influences and connecting with others who share your goals enhances your commitment to long-term success.

Finally, plan for social events and holidays. These occasions often involve food and can pose challenges to weight maintenance. Plan your meals and snacks in advance, choosing healthier options, and practice mindful eating, paying attention to your body's signals. Don't deprive yourself completely; enjoy the occasion in moderation, remembering that one meal or event won't derail your long-term progress. Focus on enjoying the social aspect rather than overindulging in food.

The journey towards a healthy weight is not a sprint, but a marathon. The long-term success lies in creating sustainable habits and making conscious choices that support your well-being, not in restrictive diets or quick fixes. By embracing mindful eating, consistent exercise, effective stress management, sufficient sleep, and a supportive community, you can confidently maintain your weight loss and enjoy a healthier, happier life. Remember that setbacks are opportunities for learning and readjustment. The ultimate goal is a sustainable lifestyle that promotes both physical and mental well-being. This is your journey, own it.

Staying Accountable and Motivated

Maintaining your weight loss isn't about unwavering rigidity; it's about cultivating a flexible, adaptable relationship with food and your body. The strategies that propelled you through the initial weight loss phase—focused meal planning, meticulous tracking—while helpful initially, may become unsustainable and even counterproductive in the long run. The key to lasting success lies in shifting your focus from strict adherence to a plan to conscious, mindful living.

This transition requires a subtle yet significant shift in mindset. Instead of viewing food as the enemy, begin to appreciate it as fuel for your body and a source of pleasure. Remember the joy you experienced discovering new recipes and flavors during your weight loss journey? Now is the time to expand upon that, to explore new culinary avenues within the framework of your chosen dietary approach—whether it's predominantly Carnivore, Paleo, or a balanced blend. Experiment with different cuts of meat, explore diverse spices and herbs, and learn to prepare meals in ways that delight your senses. This mindful approach transforms eating from a chore into a pleasurable experience, making it far more sustainable in the long run.

One effective technique for maintaining accountability is the practice of regular self-reflection. Set aside time each week—even just 15-20 minutes—to honestly assess your progress. This isn't about beating yourself up over minor slip-ups; it's about identifying patterns and making necessary adjustments. Ask yourself questions like: Am I consistently prioritizing sleep? How's my stress level? Am I incorporating enough movement into my daily routine? Are my meals satisfying and enjoyable? Honest introspection will pinpoint areas needing attention, allowing you to proactively address potential challenges before they derail your progress.

Journaling can be an invaluable tool in this self-reflection process. Record your meals, noting not only what you ate but also how you felt before, during, and after eating. Did you feel truly satisfied? Were you rushed, stressed, or emotionally eating? Identifying these triggers is crucial for preventing future impulsive choices. Similarly, document your physical activity, sleep patterns, and any stressors you encountered. Looking back on your journal entries over time reveals patterns and insights that may not be immediately apparent.

Regular weigh-ins, while important, shouldn't be the sole measure of your success. Instead of fixating on the number on the scale, consider other indicators of well-being. How are your energy levels? How's your sleep quality? Has your mood improved? These holistic metrics provide a more comprehensive picture of your overall health and progress. Focus on these positive changes, as they serve as powerful reinforcement for continuing your healthy lifestyle.

Maintaining motivation requires continuous engagement and a sense of purpose. Connect with others who share similar goals. This could involve joining online support groups, attending local fitness classes, or simply sharing your journey with friends and family. The camaraderie and encouragement from a supportive community can provide much-needed motivation when faced with challenges.

Remember, setbacks are inevitable. There will be days when you stray from your plan, and that's perfectly okay. The key is not to let these slip-ups derail your progress entirely.

Instead, acknowledge the lapse, learn from it, and move forward. Don't engage in self-criticism; view it as a temporary detour, not a complete failure. Forgive yourself and refocus on your goals. A single indulgence doesn't undo all the hard work you've accomplished.

To enhance your long-term commitment, consider setting new goals that build upon your weight loss success. Perhaps you want to improve your fitness level by participating in a 5k race, or maybe you're aiming to learn a new cooking skill. Setting achievable, yet challenging, goals provides continuous motivation and a sense of accomplishment. These goals can be related to fitness, nutrition, or personal growth; the important factor is that they align with your overall well-being and provide a sense of ongoing progress.

Visual aids can significantly enhance motivation and accountability. Create a vision board illustrating your fitness aspirations, healthy meals, and desired lifestyle. Place this board in a visible location—your refrigerator, bathroom mirror, or workstation—as a constant reminder of your goals. You can also use progress charts or apps to visually track your achievements; seeing the progress you've made can be incredibly motivating.

Consider enlisting the help of a professional. A registered dietitian or nutritionist can offer personalized guidance on maintaining a healthy, balanced diet, while a personal trainer can help you design an exercise program tailored to your fitness level and goals. Their expertise and support can be invaluable during the maintenance phase, providing you with structure and accountability.

Regular physical activity is not merely about burning calories; it's about fostering a healthy lifestyle, reducing stress, and boosting your overall well-being. Incorporate activities you genuinely enjoy—whether it's dancing, hiking, swimming, or team sports. Aim for consistency rather than intensity; regular moderate-intensity exercise is more sustainable than sporadic high-intensity workouts.

Prioritize sleep. Adequate sleep is critical for regulating hormones that control appetite and metabolism. Aim for 7-9 hours of quality sleep each night. Establish a regular sleep schedule, create a relaxing bedtime routine, and ensure your bedroom is dark, quiet, and cool.

Manage stress effectively. Chronic stress can lead to overeating and weight gain. Find healthy coping mechanisms for stress, such as meditation, yoga, spending time in nature, or engaging in hobbies. Learn to identify your stressors and develop strategies to mitigate their impact on your overall well-being.

Remember, maintaining your weight loss is a journey, not a destination. It requires ongoing commitment and adaptation. Celebrate your successes, learn from setbacks, and continuously adjust your strategies as needed. By focusing on sustainable lifestyle changes, you can confidently maintain your weight loss and live a healthier, happier life.

Embrace the process of continuous learning and improvement. There will always be new information and approaches to discover. Stay informed about the latest research on nutrition and weight management, but remember to filter the information critically and focus on evidence-based practices. Explore different approaches to exercise and nutrition, finding what works best for your individual needs and preferences.

Finally, remember that this is your journey. There's no one-size-fits-all approach; what works for one person may not work for another. Be patient with yourself, celebrate your progress, and don't be afraid to adapt your strategies as needed. The ultimate goal is to create a lifestyle that supports your long-term health and well-being, not to adhere rigidly to a specific plan. By embracing flexibility, self-compassion, and continuous self-reflection, you can achieve sustainable weight loss and maintain a healthy lifestyle for years to come. Your commitment to yourself is the most powerful tool you possess.

Making the CarnivorePaleo Lifestyle a Part of Your Life

The transition from the initial weight loss phase to long-term maintenance requires a shift in mindset. You've successfully navigated the initial challenges, learning to listen to your body's hunger cues and recognizing the satisfying fullness that comes from nutrient-dense, whole foods. Now, it's time to integrate the Carnivore-Paleo principles into your everyday life seamlessly, making them a sustainable part of your lifestyle rather than a temporary diet. This isn't about strict adherence to a rigid plan but about creating a flexible, adaptable framework for healthy eating and living.

One of the most crucial aspects of long-term success is mindful eating. This means paying attention to your body's signals – hunger, fullness, satisfaction – and responding appropriately. Avoid mindless eating, such as snacking while watching TV or eating quickly while rushing through your day. Instead, take the time to savor your meals, appreciating the textures, flavors, and aromas of your food. This mindful approach helps you connect with your body's needs and prevents overeating.

Meal preparation is another critical component of maintaining your weight loss. While you may have relied on meticulously planned meals during the initial phase, transitioning to a more flexible approach is key for long-term sustainability. Instead of rigidly adhering to a specific meal plan, focus on stocking your kitchen with Carnivore-Paleo friendly staples. This means having a variety of high-quality protein sources readily available: grass-fed beef, wild-caught fish, free-range poultry, and organic eggs. Keep your refrigerator and freezer stocked with these essentials to easily assemble quick and satisfying meals. Prepare larger batches of simple dishes on the weekends, such as roasted vegetables (if incorporating them into your plan) or a big pot of bone broth, to make weekday meal preparation easier and less time-consuming.

The beauty of the Carnivore-Paleo approach is its simplicity. It's about focusing on real, whole foods—minimizing processed ingredients and avoiding sugary drinks and refined carbohydrates. This simplicity naturally reduces the likelihood of overconsumption of calories, and the high protein and fat content contribute to sustained satiety, reducing the temptation to constantly snack. However, this doesn't mean you should deprive yourself. Allow for occasional indulgences, but practice moderation and mindfulness. A small piece of dark chocolate or a single serving of your favorite nuts (if included in your plan) can satisfy cravings without derailing your progress. The key is balance and moderation, ensuring these treats don't become frequent occurrences that counteract your efforts.

Maintaining hydration is often overlooked, yet it's crucial for overall health and weight management. Water plays a vital role in numerous bodily functions, including metabolism, digestion, and satiety. Adequate hydration can also help curb cravings, as thirst is sometimes mistaken for hunger. Aim to drink plenty of water throughout the day, and consider adding electrolyte supplements, especially if following a strict Carnivore diet, to maintain electrolyte balance. Electrolyte imbalances can lead to fatigue, muscle cramps, and other symptoms that can make it harder to stick to your plan.

Sleep is another often underestimated aspect of weight management. Chronic sleep deprivation disrupts hormone regulation, impacting appetite and metabolic rate.

Insufficient sleep can lead to increased cravings for high-calorie, sugary foods, making it more challenging to maintain your weight loss. Prioritize sleep by establishing a consistent sleep schedule, creating a relaxing bedtime routine, and ensuring your bedroom is dark, quiet, and cool. Aim for 7-9 hours of quality sleep each night. If you struggle with sleep, consider consulting a healthcare professional to rule out any underlying sleep disorders.

Incorporating regular physical activity is essential not only for weight management but also for overall health and well-being. Choose activities you genuinely enjoy—whether it's brisk walking, weight training, swimming, hiking, or any other form of movement that gets you up and moving. The key is consistency; aim for at least 150 minutes of moderate-intensity or 75 minutes of vigorous-intensity aerobic activity per week, along with strength training exercises twice a week. Remember that exercise doesn't have to be strenuous; even short bursts of activity throughout the day, such as taking the stairs instead of the elevator or going for a walk during your lunch break, can contribute to your overall fitness level.

Building a supportive community can make a significant difference in your long-term success. Connecting with others who share similar goals and challenges can provide encouragement, accountability, and a sense of belonging. Consider joining online forums, support groups, or local fitness classes to connect with like-minded individuals. Sharing your experiences, challenges, and successes with others can help you stay motivated and accountable, especially during challenging times. Don't be afraid to seek support from friends, family, or a healthcare professional when needed.

Tracking your progress is another useful tool for maintaining your weight loss. While you might have meticulously tracked every calorie and macronutrient during the initial weight loss phase, you can adopt a more relaxed approach over time. Instead of focusing solely on numbers, pay attention to how you feel – your energy levels, sleep quality, and overall well-being. Weigh yourself periodically, but don't get overly fixated on daily fluctuations. Focus on long-term trends, and celebrate your achievements along the way. Regularly reviewing your progress, whether through weight measurements, body composition analysis, or simply noting how your clothes fit, helps you stay motivated and informed about the positive changes you're making.

Social gatherings and eating out can present challenges to maintaining a Carnivore-Paleo lifestyle. However, planning ahead can make it easier to navigate these social situations. When eating out, choose restaurants that offer options compatible with your dietary preferences, such as steak houses or seafood restaurants. If you're uncertain about the ingredients in a dish, don't hesitate to ask the server about the preparation methods and ingredients. Be prepared to politely decline dishes that don't align with your dietary choices and offer alternatives. Remember that a single deviation from your plan won't derail your progress. The key is to maintain overall consistency.

It's also crucial to remember that setbacks are a normal part of the process. Don't beat yourself up over occasional slips. Instead, acknowledge them, learn from them, and move on. Focus on your overall progress and celebrate your successes, no matter how small they may seem. Maintaining a positive mindset, focusing on self-compassion, and adapting your approach as needed are essential for long-term success. Remember that this is a journey, not a race. Be patient with yourself and celebrate your achievements along the way.

Finally, remember that flexibility is key to long-term success. The Carnivore-Paleo approach isn't a rigid diet but a lifestyle. Allow for flexibility and seasonal variations in your food choices, adjusting your approach as your needs and preferences evolve. As you become more comfortable with this way of eating, you'll likely find yourself making intuitive food choices that align with the core principles of the Carnivore-Paleo lifestyle. This intuitive eating approach allows you to maintain your weight loss effortlessly, making it a sustainable part of your life for years to come. The focus shifts from strict rules to a conscious, mindful connection with your body and your food. This mindful approach empowers you to make sustainable choices that support your overall health and wellbeing. Your journey towards a healthier, happier you is ongoing – embrace the process and enjoy the benefits.

Celebrating Your Success

You've done it. You've reached a significant milestone on your journey towards a healthier, happier you. The weight loss you've achieved is a testament to your commitment, discipline, and unwavering dedication. This isn't just about the numbers on the scale; it's about the positive changes you've experienced in your energy levels, sleep quality, and overall well-being. Celebrate this achievement! You deserve it.

Don't underestimate the power of acknowledging your accomplishments. This isn't about vanity; it's about reinforcing positive behavior and motivating yourself to continue on this path. Take time to reflect on how far you've come. Think back to the beginning of your journey. Remember those initial challenges, the moments of doubt, and the times you felt like giving up. Now, look at how far you've progressed. This reflection is crucial for bolstering your confidence and reinforcing the positive changes you've made.

How can you celebrate your success? The best celebrations are those that align with your new, healthier lifestyle. Instead of indulging in sugary treats or high-carbohydrate meals, consider these rewarding alternatives:

Treat yourself to a new piece of workout gear:
Investing in new athletic wear or a fitness gadget can serve as a
motivational reminder of your commitment to your health and fitness goals. A new pair of comfortable walking shoes or a heart rate monitor can make your workouts more enjoyable and effective. Consider a new yoga mat, resistance

bands, or a kettlebell – anything that inspires you to continue your fitness routine.

Enjoy a luxurious bath or massage:
Pamper yourself with a relaxing bath infused with essential oils, or indulge in a professional massage. These experiences promote relaxation and stress reduction, which are essential for maintaining a healthy weight. Stress often leads to unhealthy eating habits, so reducing stress is a crucial part of long-term weight
management.

Go on a hike or nature walk:
Spend time in nature. A scenic hike or nature walk provides exercise, fresh air, and a chance to appreciate the beauty of the outdoors. This is a much healthier way to celebrate than indulging in unhealthy foods.

Take a photography class:
Learn a new skill and engage your mind creatively. This is a fantastic way to invest in personal growth, reduce stress, and shift your focus from food-based rewards. Learning a new skill builds confidence and provides a sense of accomplishment, further reinforcing your successful weight loss journey.

Plan a special healthy meal:
Instead of celebratory foods that derail your progress, focus on preparing a delicious and nutritious meal featuring high-quality ingredients. This could be a beautifully plated steak with roasted asparagus and a side salad, or a pan-seared salmon with vibrant vegetables. The key is to savor the delicious flavors of the meal, mindful of its nutritional benefits. This reinforces healthy eating habits and demonstrates how delicious and satisfying a Carnivore-Paleo lifestyle can be.

Buy a new book or subscribe to an inspiring podcast:
Expand your knowledge and cultivate self-improvement.

This helps to maintain a positive mindset and keeps you engaged in your personal growth. Investing in self-improvement promotes mental well-being, which is another significant factor in long-term weight management.

Spend quality time with loved ones:
Connect with friends and family in meaningful ways. Social connection
contributes to happiness and overall well-being, helping to prevent stress-induced eating. Sharing your success story with your support system can also be incredibly rewarding.

Beyond these specific suggestions, remember that the best celebration is one that genuinely reflects your personal values and interests. It's about reinforcing the positive changes you've made and setting the stage for continued success. Avoid celebrations that undo your hard work – that's counterproductive. Focus on activities that promote well-being, strengthen your commitment, and bring you joy.

Maintaining your weight loss long-term is about more than just the food you eat; it's about establishing sustainable lifestyle habits. Celebrating your milestones along the way is a vital part of this process. It helps to solidify your commitment and create positive reinforcement for continuing your journey.

Sustaining Your Momentum: Beyond the Celebration

Now that you've celebrated your success, let's talk about maintaining the momentum. The journey doesn't end here; this is an ongoing commitment to your health and well-being. Think of your weight loss as a marathon, not a sprint. Maintaining your weight loss requires consistent effort and mindful attention to your lifestyle.

Continue Tracking Your Progress:
Don't stop tracking your food intake, even if you've reached your goal weight.
This will help you stay mindful of your eating habits and identify any potential triggers for weight gain. However, the focus now shifts from strict tracking to more mindful awareness of your food choices.

Adjust Your Caloric Intake:
As you maintain your weight, your caloric needs may change. Pay attention to your body's hunger cues and adjust your food intake accordingly. You might find that your appetite naturally adjusts to a slightly lower or higher calorie intake compared to the initial weight-loss phase.

Stay Active:
Exercise remains crucial for maintaining your weight loss. Find activities you genuinely enjoy, and stick with them. Consistency is key. Aim for at least 150 minutes of moderate-intensity exercise or 75 minutes of vigorous-intensity exercise per week, along with strength training exercises at least twice a week.

Prioritize Sleep:
Adequate sleep is essential for weight management. Aim for 7-9 hours of quality sleep each night.
Sleep deprivation can disrupt hormones that regulate appetite, potentially leading to increased hunger and cravings.

Manage Stress:
Stress can lead to unhealthy eating habits. Find healthy ways to manage stress, such as meditation, yoga, spending time in nature, or engaging in hobbies you enjoy.

Stay Hydrated:
Drink plenty of water throughout the day.
Water helps to keep you feeling full, aids digestion, and supports overall bodily functions. Staying properly hydrated is crucial for a healthy metabolism and overall well-being.

Dealing with Plateaus and Setbacks

It's normal to encounter plateaus or even experience occasional setbacks on your weight-loss journey. Don't let these discourage you. Plateaus are a natural part of the process, and setbacks are opportunities for learning and growth.

If you hit a plateau, re-evaluate your diet and exercise routine. Are you consuming enough protein? Are you getting sufficient electrolytes? Are you consistently following your chosen exercise plan? Consider making minor adjustments to your approach to break through the plateau. For example, you may need to slightly increase your exercise intensity or adjust your macronutrient ratios.

Setbacks can happen. Perhaps you indulged in a less-than-ideal meal, or you missed a few workouts. Don't beat yourself up about it! Acknowledge the setback, learn from it, and get back on track as soon as possible. This is about making progress, not perfection. The key is to remain committed to your long-term goals and adjust your strategy as needed.

The Power of Mindset: Embracing Long-Term Success

Maintaining your weight loss is largely a mental game. It's about developing a healthy relationship with food and exercise and adopting a mindset of sustainable lifestyle changes. The Carnivore-Paleo approach isn't just a diet; it's a lifestyle shift that promotes long-term health and well-being. Remember that flexibility and adaptability are key. You don't have to be perfect; you just have to be consistent in your efforts to make healthy choices the majority of the time.

Develop a strong support system. Share your journey with friends, family, or a support group. Having people who understand your goals and encourage your progress can make a significant difference. Accountability is powerful – consider partnering with someone else who shares similar goals.

Celebrate your non-scale victories as well. Focus on improvements in your energy levels, sleep quality, mental clarity, and overall well-being. These are equally important indicators of success.

Remember, your journey towards a healthier lifestyle is ongoing. There will be ups and downs, but by celebrating your successes, learning from setbacks, and maintaining a positive mindset, you can achieve long-term weight loss and maintain a healthier, happier you for years to come. This isn't a temporary fix; this is a sustainable change for a lifetime of better health. Embrace the process and enjoy the journey. You've earned it.

Acknowledgments

First and foremost, I want to express my sincere gratitude to all the individuals who have supported me throughout the writing of this book. This includes my family and friends for their unwavering patience and encouragement, especially during those late nights spent researching and writing. A special thanks goes to [Name of editor/agent, if applicable], whose insightful feedback and expertise significantly enhanced the clarity and impact of the manuscript.

I also want to acknowledge the countless individuals who have shared their personal experiences with the Carnivore and Paleo diets. Your stories of success, resilience, and transformation have been an invaluable source of inspiration and motivation. Your willingness to share your journeys has helped shape this book's practical approach and empathetic tone. Finally, my gratitude extends to the medical professionals and researchers whose work has informed my understanding of nutrition and weight management. Their contributions to the scientific community have provided the foundation for the evidence-based advice presented within these pages.

Appendix

This appendix provides additional resources to support your Carnivore-Paleo journey.

Appendix A: Detailed Macronutrient Breakdown of Sample Recipes:

This section provides a comprehensive breakdown of the macronutrient content (protein, fat, and carbohydrates) for each recipe included in Chapter 3.

Appendix B: Sample Weekly Shopping Lists:

Several sample weekly shopping lists are provided to help you plan your grocery shopping efficiently. These lists are categorized based on different levels of dietary adherence and budget considerations.

Appendix C: Conversion Charts:

Useful conversion charts are included for measurements, including ounces to grams, cups to milliliters, etc.

Appendix D: List of Recommended Supplements:

A list of supplements that may be beneficial for those following a Carnivore-Paleo diet, along with considerations for usage and potential interactions. It's important to note that this is not exhaustive, and individual needs vary significantly. Always consult with your healthcare provider before starting any supplement regimen.

Glossary

Basal Metabolic Rate (BMR):
The number of calories your body burns at rest to maintain basic functions.

Calorie Deficit:
Consuming fewer calories than your body expends, leading to weight loss.

Carnivore Diet:
A dietary approach that primarily consists of animal products, such as meat, fish, and eggs.

Glycemic Index (GI):
A ranking system for carbohydrates based on how quickly they raise blood sugar levels.

HIIT (High-Intensity Interval Training):
A form of exercise characterized by short bursts of intense activity followed by periods of rest or low-intensity activity.

Insulin Resistance:
A condition in which the body's cells become less responsive to insulin, leading to elevated blood sugar levels.

Ketogenic Diet:
A very low-carbohydrate, high-fat diet that forces the body to enter a metabolic state called ketosis, where it burns fat for energy instead of glucose.

Macronutrients:
The three main components of food: carbohydrates, proteins, and fats.

Paleo Diet:
A dietary approach based on the foods believed to have
been eaten by our ancestors during the Paleolithic era.

Thermic Effect of Food (TEF):
The number of calories your body burns to digest, absorb, and metabolize food.

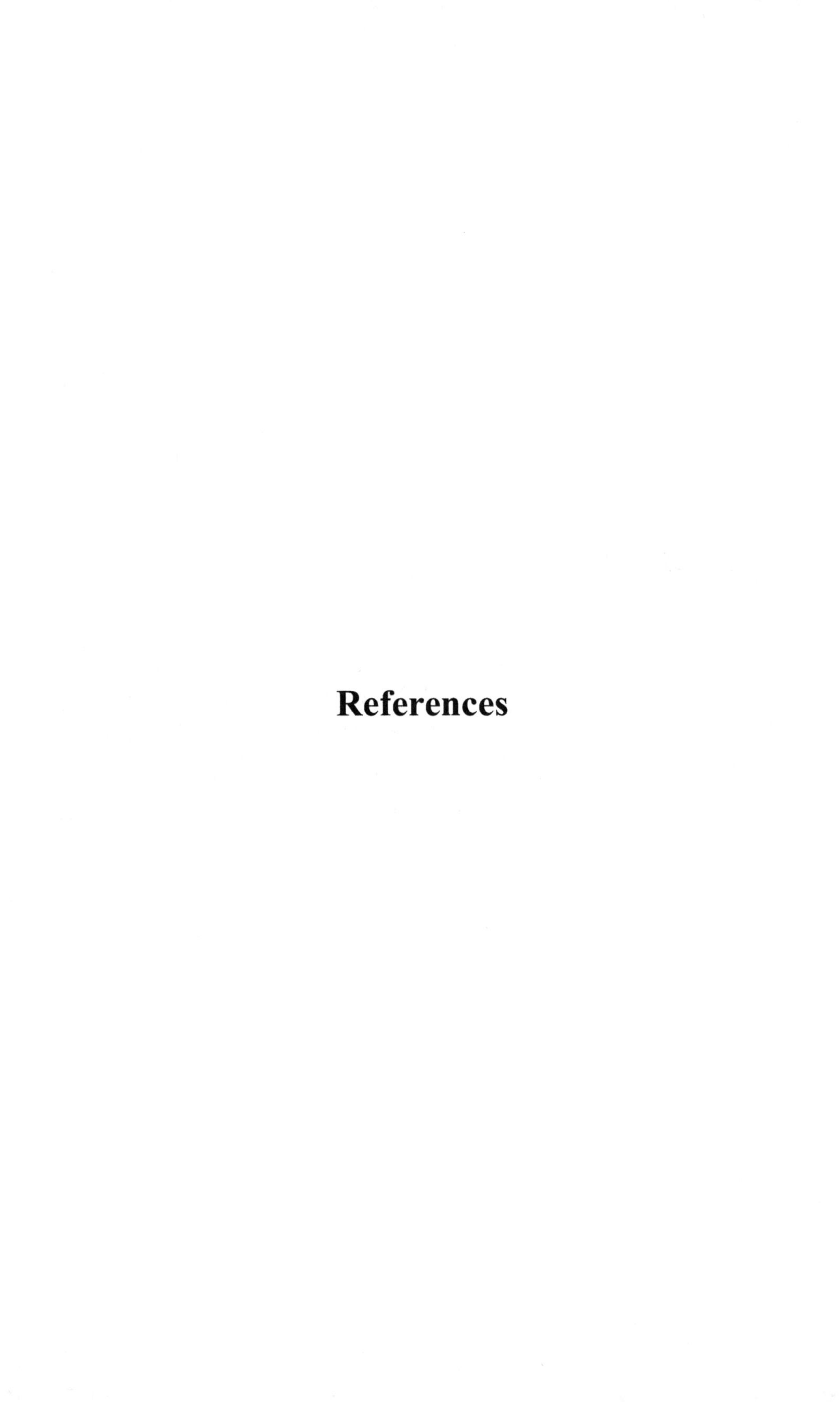

References

Author Biography

Scott Johnsey has spent most of his adult life studying and researching all of the diet and exercise routines through the years. He has combed through everything from fad diets to medical research. This book brings out the most common sense approach to weight loss and exercise that he fills can be implemented and continually successful for life.